CANCER ON THE MARGINS:
METHOD AND MEANING IN PARTICIPATORY RESEARCH

Cancer on the Margins presents the findings of the Ontario Breast Cancer Community Research Initiative, an organization created to investigate the experiences of women with breast cancer from marginalized and underrepresented groups. The authors examine the psychosocial needs of women living with breast cancer, while investigating differences in treatment, care, and survivorship among Aboriginal women, women of colour, Francophone women, lesbians, as well as young women, lower-income women, and women in rural areas.

Structured as a guide for similar research, *Cancer on the Margins* provides a 'start to finish' format that reveals the complexities of doing such work at each stage, beginning with the study design and ending with the dissemination of results. The authors address the issues of working with and speaking for these groups of women, the tension between description and interpretation, and the challenge for qualitative work to present findings that positively influence the circumstances of research participants. With a strong commitment to social justice, this volume shows how participatory research can lead to social change and indicates effective ways to ensure that research not only reaches but is also employed in the communities it intends to serve.

Bridging the gap between a wide range of audiences, this vitally important work will be of interest to health professionals, policy makers, new researchers, and experienced investigators, as well as the public.

JENNIFER J. NELSON is an independent research consultant and an assistant professor in the Department of Public Health Sciences at the University of Toronto.

JUDY GOULD is a research scientist at Women's College Research Institute and an assistant professor in the Department of Public Health Sciences at the University of Toronto.

SUE KELLER-OLAMAN is an adjunct professor in the Department of Health, Aging and Society at McMaster University.

T0219256

EDITED BY JENNIFER J. NELSON, JUDY GOULD,
AND SUE KELLER-OLAMAN

Cancer on the Margins

Method and Meaning in Participatory Research

UNIVERSITY OF TORONTO PRESS
Toronto Buffalo London

© University of Toronto Press Incorporated 2009
Toronto Buffalo London
www.utppublishing.com
Printed in Canada

ISBN 978-0-8020-9169-7 (cloth)
ISBN 978-0-8020-9434-6 (paper)

Library and Archives Canada Cataloguing in Publication

Cancer on the margins : method and meaning in participatory research /
edited by Jennifer J. Nelson, Judy Gould, and Sue Keller-Olaman.

Includes bibliographical references and index.
ISBN 978-0-8020-9169-7 (bound). – ISBN 978-0-8020-9434-6 (pbk.)

1. Breast – Cancer – Patients – Ontario – Social conditions – Research.
2. Cancer in women – Social aspects – Research – Ontario.   3. Women –
Health and hygiene – Research – Ontario.   4. Women – Medical care –
Research – Ontario.   5. Participant observation.   I. Nelson, Jennifer J.
(Jennifer Jill), 1972– .   II. Gould, Judy, 1966– .   III. Keller-Olaman, Sue

RC267.C3646 2009   362.196′9944900720713   C2008–907898–5

University of Toronto Press acknowledges the financial assistance to its
publishing program of the Canada Council for the Arts and the Ontario
Arts Council.

University of Toronto Press acknowledges the financial support for its
publishing activities of the Government of Canada through the Book
Publishing Industry Development Program (BPIDP).

Contents

PART FIVE: IMPLICATIONS AND IMPACTS OF KNOWLEDGE

List of Tables

Foreword

This book is the culmination of a six-year program of participatory, psychosocial research in the field of breast cancer in Ontario, Canada. The research program emerged through a commitment by the Canadian Breast Cancer Foundation, Ontario Chapter (CBCF, ON) to make a difference in the daily lives of women diagnosed with breast cancer by funding research that honoured the experience and wisdom of these women, their loved ones, and those health professionals and volunteers who support them. CBCF, ON approached the Centre for Research in Women's Health, a partnership of the University of Toronto and Women's College Hospital, to develop a new research unit with this focus in mind. In partnership with Drs. Ross Gray and Marg Fitch, two respected investigators from the Psychosocial and Behavioural Research Unit of Toronto Sunnybrook Regional Cancer Centre, the Ontario Breast Cancer Community Research Initiative (OBCCRI) was created.

The initiative had a particular commitment to reach women who might not normally be heard – women scraping by on low incomes, women of colour, Aboriginal women, older women, immigrant women, to name a few – in order to add their voices to the chorus of others who want to insure optimal quality of life and optimal quality of services for women during this deeply challenging period of their lives.

In addition to using participatory research approaches, the Unit had two other objectives: to mentor new researchers in order to create a larger cadre of individuals with expertise in community-based research, and to focus on innovative methods of dissemination so that the learnings would be put to use – to enhance quality of life and to improve cancer support services.

It is with a great sense of pride that I write the foreword to this book.

This book captures, for others who want to use community-based and participatory approaches, the processes, dilemmas, challenges, and pleasures of working in this paradigm. These relatively new investigators, along with their research assistants and project advisors, have matured to such a degree that they have, literally, a book full of thoughtful and provocative insights. They attend to questions of who deserves to be heard, who is able to speak for whom, whether the researcher can speak for herself, and if so, under what circumstances. They query the tricky questions of unequal power in academic/community partnerships, in intellectual versus experiential discourses, and in dominant versus non-dominant cultures. They illustrate, using case studies, possibilities for improved research practice – how to transcend the 'research chill' that has emerged in communities where research 'on' or research 'for' has taken precedence over research 'with.'

Issues of trust are examined, as are issues of reciprocity. There are some wonderful depictions of the complexity of the analytic process, which concretize the type of thinking that yields thick versus thin or layered versus simplistic interpretations. The fraught role of interpreter or narrator is examined at length, as is the question of the attention paid to contexts, both micro and macro.

Ultimately, the authors converge on their fundamental commitment to social justice for women with breast cancer. They start with issues of engagement, authenticity, power and privilege, trust, voice, and reciprocity, and end with a plea for inclusion, equity, and empowerment. None of these ideas is unproblematic. But the chapters in this book shine with intelligence, thoughtfulness, commitment, humility, and grace. In the final analysis, I have concluded, it is these traits, more than any others, that augur for the successful implementation of research 'with' our community partners.

Heather Maclean
Vice-President of Research and Inter-Professional Education
Women's College Hospital, Toronto

Acknowledgments

The editors would like to extend our sincere thanks to the many individuals and organizations who have made this book possible. The Canadian Breast Cancer Foundation, Ontario Chapter, supported the research initiative with infrastructure funding from 2001 to 2007, as well as funding various individual studies. We are very grateful to Manon Labrecque, our research assistant, and Angela Sardelis, our research secretary, who provided phenomenal office support throughout the research initiative and the production of this book. We also appreciate the excellent work of Jiji Voronka during the early phases of the book's conceptualization. Mary Newberry, our copy editor, has been instrumental in bringing the book to fruition, and we appreciate her exquisite attention to detail. We are very grateful to the staff at University of Toronto Press for many hours of fine work. Stephen Kotowych saw the manuscript through its earlier phases of review and acceptance. Daniel Quinlan and Wayne Herrington have seen the production through to the end. We also want to thank our three anonymous peer reviewers, whose feedback greatly strengthened the work. Certainly not least, we are extremely grateful to the women who participated in all of our research projects over the years, both as advisory committee members and as research participants. Their stories and insight are the backbone of this work.

CANCER ON THE MARGINS:
METHOD AND MEANING IN PARTICIPATORY RESEARCH

Introduction

> Not everything that can be counted counts, and not everything that counts can be counted.
>
> —Albert Einstein (*attributed*)

This wise bit of insight encapsulates much of the drive and motivation behind the research represented in this book. In some ways, it speaks to the very core of qualitative, exploratory research – that is, the need to delve underneath the statistics and 'facts' to ask critical questions about *why* things are as they seem, why things occur in a particular way, and from whose perspective, in what context, and so on. For most of us in this book who approach psychosocial issues in breast cancer care from social science backgrounds, these investigative entry points are commonplace; however, when applied in the healthcare arena, as methods to illuminate human experience and social relations, they are relatively new. We might know, for instance, how many patients experience financial problems during a cancer diagnosis, but how can we trace these stories of hardship to the specific policies and practices that underpin or exacerbate them? How do we understand something of the myriad systemic factors behind socioeconomic inequality? And what do patients themselves think about their encounters with community programs, medical professionals, or support groups? These are a few of the kinds of questions addressed in the pages of this volume.

We might even be so bold as to add to Einstein's dictum: 'not everything that counts *is counted*.' In this, we refer to marginalized forms of knowledge that have been so important to identify and consider during the research trajectory presented here. For instance, little is known about the nature of the cancer experience for women who are not middle class, white, middle aged, and heterosexual. A major impetus in our work has been to look not only at different women's experiences, but at the social forces and inequities that shape those experiences. This, too, is reflected in many of the chapters.

When we met as a group to draft a proposal for this book, we brought a variety of concerns. We wanted the book to be accessible to as many audiences as possible without losing the analytic complexity in the various studies. We also wanted to address some of the 'how to' issues that arise at different stages of the research process, like recruiting, writing ethics proposals, working with communities, and seeing that the work gets out into the world – without providing simplified 'recipes' or finite solutions.

The latter point is particularly important as, perhaps above all, we wished for the writing to inspire questions, conversations, reflections, and critical thinking about how researchers approach their subjects of inquiry. We have, therefore, endeavoured to provide something of a guide for those who might want to engage in participatory and/or community-based research. And, for those who already do such research, we offer our experiences, analyses, challenges, and lessons as points of comparison, contrast, or critique. Although no single book will resonate with all possible audiences, our hope is that different aspects of the work engage a variety of readers; undergraduate students in medicine, healthcare, and social science fields, for example, might find it a useful introduction to the kinds of questions addressed by qualitative work on health issues; graduate students might benefit from discussions that broach methodological design and the practicalities of transforming curiosity into a viable study; experienced qualitative researchers, we hope, will relate to and engage with the ethical and theoretical concerns stemming from the discussions, while those who undertake other forms of research may take interest in the relevant additional insights offered by qualitative, psychosocial work.

We hope that healthcare practitioners might benefit from the findings presented on both the patient perspectives and systemic inequalities that inform our concerns over cancer treatment and aftercare – concerns that we know practitioners not only share but confront on a much more regular and front-line basis. Patients and community advocates, we hope, might also find use for analysis that attempts to think through the challenges inherent in employing research for social change. We believe this collection has application beyond cancer care, and even beyond healthcare; at its core are questions of equality, responsibility, relationships, and ethics as they inform the search for a better understanding of illness and health.

We are aware of having posed more questions than we answer, but we think this is both part and parcel of critical, reflexive research, and that it speaks to the infeasibility of overarching solutions to research challenges. We attempt, instead, to consider the particular problems of knowledge, relationships, subject positions, methodologies, power, ethics, and social justice within their particular political, personal, and relational frameworks.

Herein, we introduce the history of our research unit and situate it within the 'landscape' in which our intellectual concerns take shape and evolve, and which we, in turn, participate in shaping.

Quick Facts

- In Ontario, in 2007, an estimated 8,500 women were diagnosed with breast cancer and 2,000 were expected to die of this disease (Canadian Cancer Society, 2007)
- In Ontario by 2001, of those who had been diagnosed during the previous 20 years, 78,528 individuals were still living (Hrabar, personal communication, 2002)
- Quality of life and supportive care issues are central concerns for women diagnosed with breast cancer (Canadian Breast Cancer Foundation, Ontario Chapter, 2006)
- Limited data exist on how people experience the breast cancer diagnosis and treatment, particularly poor women, women of colour, and Aboriginal women (Macleod et al., 2000; Ashing-Giwa & Ganz, 1997; Marrett & Chaudhry, 2003)

From the limited research that exists, we do know, for instance, that lower-income women and Aboriginal women have higher mortality rates than do middle- and upper-income women (Macleod et al., 2000; Marrett & Chaudhry, 2003), that more women under forty die of breast cancer than of any other type of cancer (Canadian Cancer Society, 2002), and that most young women have more difficulties adapting to diagnosis and treatment (Lewis et al., 2001). We know that older women's cancer treatment and their quality and length of life after a cancer diagnosis may be compromised by social factors (Lickley, 1997). And we know that lesbian breast cancer patients are less satisfied than heterosexual patients with their physicians' care and with the involvement of their partners in medical treatment (Fobair et al., 2001).

Generally, we are just beginning to understand more about how women view themselves, their illnesses, and their lives within particular social contexts. Their relayed experiences have illuminated many remaining questions – for example, about how racism, homophobia, and socioeconomic oppression function as systemic barriers to healthcare.

To address these voids, in 2001 the Canadian Breast Cancer Foundation, Ontario Chapter invested $1.7 million in the creation of an innovative research unit, the Ontario Breast Cancer Community Research Initiative (OBCCRI). This research unit was mandated to study the psychosocial needs of marginalized or underrepresented communities of women with breast cancer.

In June 2001, we at OBCCRI carried out a needs assessment with healthcare providers and survivors in the breast cancer community to guide our decisions about where to focus our research (Gray, 2002). This exercise, conducted in cooperation with the Ontario Breast Cancer Information Exchange Partnership, helped us identify the groups of women whose experiences were not well understood, while also illuminating some common needs and issues among women living with breast cancer. These findings suggested that we needed to focus particularly on understanding the breast cancer diagnosis, treatment, and survivorship experiences of the following groups:

- young women (especially those with children)
- women over seventy years old
- low-income women
- Aboriginal women
- racially marginalized women
- rural women
- lesbian/gay/bisexual/transgendered/transsexual (LGBTT) women
- Francophone women

Over the next six years, OBCCRI created a unique body of psychosocial knowledge about the experiences of women and families affected by breast cancer, with particular attention to the above groups and the issues that are central to them. From 2001 through 2007, we carried out 28 mainly qualitative and participatory research projects, stimulated new cancer support services by providing an evidence base for advocacy, presented our work to many scholarly and community audiences, and built lasting connections among caregivers, researchers, and marginalized communities. Our projects explored women's supportive care needs, their coping strategies, the community support they receive, their family situations, the resources available to them, their understanding of their disease, and their experiences with the healthcare system. Many studies placed particular emphasis on how systemic inequalities can disproportionately influence these factors for different groups, and most took a community-based approach to these issues. In particular, we addressed issues of social inequality in partnership with lower-income women, LGBTT activists, rural women, women from age groups (under forty-five and over seventy) that have been underrepresented, women of colour, and Francophone women. Studies explored the financial hardships of cancer, the effects of racism, colonialism, and homophobia on community health and support, the problems of geographic and cultural isolation, and the benefits, challenges, and particularities of supportive care. Issues of linguistic marginalization arose, unsurprisingly, in the Francophone study, but were also poignant in studies with women of colour and immigrant women, particularly with regard to accessible information materials and communication with healthcare providers.

This volume, then, draws on a number of studies from our cache, and conveys many of the issues and concerns we have identified over the years. The contributors are social scientists, students, research assistants, cancer survivor advisory group members, and associates of the research unit, all of whom bring distinct insights and points of view. Importantly, the words of our research participants, women with breast cancer, are also evident throughout.

Some studies in this volume also incorporate the experiences of participants with forms of cancer other than breast. While our central mandate was to study breast cancer, many of the issues are similar across disease sites, and some studies broadened their topics to 'women's cancers' or 'breast and gynecological cancers.' Often, a few women with other forms of cancer would volunteer to participate in a study, and we did not wish to exclude their experiences and views.

As mentioned above, we have attempted to provide guidance, examples, and critical questions that we have found relevant at each particular stage of the research process. As such, while there is much overlap throughout among the practical 'steps' of study design and the attendant theoretical and philosophical work, the book is organized somewhat 'chronologically' by research stage: it begins with the early inklings of curiosity about a topic, and moves through the formation of a research question, the design of a methodology, and the ethics approval process and its related considerations. Along the way, we discuss community engagement, the building of teams and relationships, and the intricacies of working with others across different social positions and power imbalances. These foundational considerations give way to the analytic process –in other words, once we have collected the data, how do we make sense of it? And analysis is followed closely by and intricately bound up with discussions of the representation of findings – in other words, once we think we have an analysis, how do we talk and write about it, and what do we need to think about while doing so? On a related note, we move to some critical reflection on the researcher's role in knowledge production and the roles of other research team members, all of which illustrate the personal commitments, investments, concerns, and blind spots that merit our attention as they affect the work we do. The final chapters of the book are concerned with the later stages of the research process – the meanings, methods, benefits, tensions, and risks of putting knowledge 'out there,' to be employed in concrete practices and processes.

Within the chapters, we have provided, at the first mention, short tables summarizing each research project. These are intended to offer a basic sense of the projects 'at a glance.' While many chapters present more in-depth data from the various projects, the focus, in most cases, is on the processes behind the research at specific phases – the concerns, challenges, lessons, or questions that arose for the authors, their teams, and their participants.

Part one, Research Design in Participatory Approaches, illustrates initial considerations and processes of engagement with communities as research gets off the ground. In the first chapter, Sue Keller-Olaman and Stephanie Austin provide an accessible, hands-on introduction to setting up a research project for those who may be new to community-based work. With examples of key methodological and ethical issues from their own work, they set the stage for the rest of the chapters by laying out foundational concepts: they clearly distinguish qualitative from quantitative philosophies, define participatory approaches and some common methodologies, and discuss the selection of appropriate methods according to the researcher's particular interests and curiosities. This groundwork acquaints the reader with several preoccupations that run throughout the book: questions as to the authorship of data, the involvement of communities, the importance of relationships, the politics of social and power differences, and the need for research-driven activism.

In chapter 2, Stephanie Austin zeroes in on ethical issues from a few different angles. On a philosophical level, she considers what it means to plan projects that are relevant and responsive to community needs. Politically, she is concerned with equity and working across differences in ways that do not replicate oppressive research practices. At the same time, she addresses the practicalities of ethical considerations – the formal ethics review process, confidentiality, the careful use of project funds, and tensions around matching community and academic resources and interests. Drawing on her work with Francophone women, Austin broadens 'ethics' to encompass questions about personal and professional integrity, political goals, and a commitment to equality in collaborative work.

In chapter 3, Terry Mitchell and Emerance Baker continue the dialogue about what it means to do ethical research – in their case, with Aboriginal communities. As a Native and a non-Native researcher, they discuss the experiences and challenges of engaging with Native communities in a participatory action research project. The authors attend to the historical colonial context in which research about Aboriginal groups has developed, and to the understandable 'research chill' that has resulted as communities reassess and reclaim control over outsiders' access to and authorship of their lives. As an example of this reclamation, they discuss the principles of 'ownership, control, access, and possession' of research data, which are increasingly defining ethics processes in research by and with Aboriginal communities. Like Austin, ethics is, for these authors, as much about self-reflexive accounting for subjectivity and historical context as it is about building respectful relationships and attending to a balance of researcher and community benefits.

Part two, Approaches in Data Analysis, comprises two reflective chapters that tackle the daunting issues we as researchers face around what to do with our reams of data once it is collected. In chapter 4, Judy Gould, Chris Sinding, Terry Mitchell, and Margaret I. Fitch provide us with a map of their analytic journey across three separate studies under the umbrella of a larger research project. As they approach the task of thinking both individually and collectively about their findings, they also attend to the challenges and benefits of 'thinking with' various project teams and several communities of women at once. This leads them to forge an innovative method for critically considering how different perspectives and experiences both resonate and contrast with one another, while keeping in mind the complexities and intersections of identities.

In chapter 5, Chris Sinding tells the story of grappling with two different analytic approaches to her interviews with caregivers looking after loved ones who had cancer. Although both were generated within grounded theory methodology, each approach, she makes clear, took her down a different road, leading to new questions and some surprising angles from which to view her findings. Sinding's intricate description of her choices around how to think about, code, and interpret her findings offers a concrete demonstration of the complexities – and responsibilities – of meaning making.

Part three, The Politics of Representation, urges us to ask critical questions about what it means to speak of others' lives, often across key political and social inequalities, and within the philosophical dimensions of research that draws on community-based and participatory approaches. In chapter 6, Chris Sinding, Lisa Barnoff, Pamela Grassau, Fran Odette, and Patti McGillicuddy struggle over the tensions around which voices and issues to emphasize, and which data best express the experiences of their participants. They consider what, when, and how to 'strategically essentialize' – to highlight certain findings or analyses according to the specificities of audience, context, and goals. They walk a difficult line, negotiating competing demands within the same community and participant group, but always maintaining the integrity of the collective research process; in this, they demonstrate the strengths of this process not only for defining and shaping project goals, but for working out difficult analytic questions and making space for divergent claims.

Jennifer J. Nelson, in chapter 7, takes up similar issues, grappling with how to portray the voices of women of colour in light of her political concerns about how they might be heard in some audiences and disciplines. She considers her own problematic position as researcher within systems of domination and marginality. She draws on the methods of Michel Foucault to make connections between knowledge and power, and to critically consider the risks around knowledge production that leave the implications of authorship unnamed.

All the authors in this section depict their efforts to make transparent the necessary process of decision-making that is often obscured in research accounts, while also remaining true to participants' meanings, embedded as they are within complex sets of power relations.

Part four, Reflections on Research: From Different Standpoints, entails something of a departure from the process of research itself, although its deliberations are, we believe, integral. Here, several authors take a step outside the bounds of our projects and, from various points of view, think back on our own roles and positions as researchers and team members. The authors are concerned with how subject positions, power differentials, life experiences, and various kinds of connection and disconnection with research participants can serve, variously, as potential blind spots or useful points of understanding. Above all, they are concerned with how these factors can shape the research and its outcomes in ways that are not always apparent. Without providing hard and fast tenets, these chapters illustrate the need for critical reflection throughout the research process – reflection on who we think we are as researchers/activists/team members constitutes not only the beliefs and biases we bring to the issues, but how we relate to participants, the kind of knowledge we produce, and how it might be mobilized in our project sites.

In chapter 8, Jennifer J. Nelson and Judy Gould think through their positions as principal investigators vis-à-vis the communities with whom they work. Through excerpts from a transcribed conversation, they ponder the influence of personal histories on their current research choices, and the intricacies of their shifting subject positions over time. They describe how the particularities or small moments of disruption in a research process are often most telling of the larger dynamics of power that encase knowledge production. They discuss ways in which subjectivity influences not only choices of research area, but also the relationships with participants and the resulting analysis. Through these considerations, they explore the meaning and fluidity of subjectivity itself, the traps of essentialism, and the ever-present need to ground the issues and relationships at hand in the larger historical and socio-political contexts through which they have developed.

Pamela Grassau and Kara Griffin, in chapter 9, offer insights into the research process from a perspective that is not often represented in methodological and reflective accounts – that of the graduate student research assistant or project coordinator. Often the overseer of relationships throughout a research process, the coordinator is tasked with thinking through the day to day needs of participants and researchers alike, yet we hear little of the influence of this role on research projects, and little of the experience of this work for those who perform it. Using the metaphor of a pathway, Grassau and Griffin offer us their perspectives on engaging with communities in meaningful, responsible, and mutually beneficial ways. They offer several themes for critical consideration – power, privilege, trust, voice, and reciprocity – illustrated through their own experiences.

Chapter 10 offers yet another set of reflections from a less visible research role. Here, Patti McGillicuddy, Falia Damianakis, Ann Wray Hampson, and Judy Gould, based on a recorded conversation, write from their perspectives as cancer survivors with professional skills and interests in psychosocial cancer issues and as advisory committee members who consult on OBCCRI research. Their comments incite us to keep research grounded in the lived struggles of communities, and remind us of the richness of an exploratory process in which various viewpoints are brought to bear. They engage in a dialogue about these and other issues such as tokenism and essentialism, as well as how they might or might not 'speak for' other cancer survivors. Finally, they provide recommendations for others who wish to engage members of their participant communities in advisory roles.

The book's final section, Implications and Impacts of Knowledge, rounds out our trajectory by considering the place of research knowledge in the communities with whom we work. Here, it becomes even more apparent that the employment of in-depth consultation and participatory processes are not simply intellectual exercises; rather, Sinding and Gould write, with OBCCRI co-founder Ross Gray, about the process of communicating findings to the communities with whom we work. With examples drawn from a research-based drama and a national OBCCRI study, they illustrate how the impacts of new knowledge can be not only far-reaching, but sometimes unexpected.

Margaret Fitch concludes our collection in chapter 12 with a comprehensive overview of the complexities of using research knowledge to effect changes in cancer care. Attending to factors such as institutional context, receptivity, target audience, relationships, and communication challenges across research paradigms, she poses essential considerations for all researchers concerned with social change. For example: By whom, for whom, and by what means should research knowledge be transferred and employed? What are the best ways to influence policy around specific issues? How does one make decisions about which directions and strategies to foreground given the limits in energy and resources? Perhaps most fundamentally, what are our expectations for 'the use of knowledge,' and what does this really mean for the future of psychosocial work?

As this final section makes clear, the need for ongoing, rigorous inquiry into the social and experiential realms of cancer, and how they might best be incorporated in health systems, is immense – and the contribution of this work, considering its brief history, already profound.

REFERENCES

Ashing-Giwa, K., & Ganz, P.A. (1997). Understanding the breast cancer experience of African-American women. *Journal of Psychosocial Oncology, 15*(2), 19–35.

Canadian Breast Cancer Foundation, Ontario Chapter. (2006). *Toward kinder care*. Retrieved November 14, 2008, from http://www.upfrontproject.ca/documents/TowardKinderCare-final.pdf

Canadian Cancer Society. (2002). Canadian Cancer Society statistics. Retrieved September 2002, from http://www.cancer.ca/files/stats2002_e.pdf

Canadian Cancer Society. (2007). Canadian Cancer Society statistics. Retrieved September 2007, from http://www.cancer.ca/ccs/internet/standard/0,3182,3543_314950__langId-en,00.html

Fobair, P., O'Hanlan, K., Koopman, C., Classen, C., Dimiceli, S., Drooker, N., Warner, D., Davids, H., Loulan, J., Wallsten, D., Goffinet, D., Morrow, G., & Spiegel, D. (2001). Comparison of lesbian and heterosexual women's response to newly diagnosed breast cancer. *Psycho-Oncology, 10*(1), 40–51.

Gray, R. (2002). *Needs and issues relevant to future breast cancer research in Ontario report*. Psychosocial and Behavioural Research Unit, Sunnybrook and Women's College Health Sciences Centre, Toronto, ON.

Lewis, J., Manne, S., DuHamel, K., Vicksburg, S., Bovbjerg, D., Currie, V., Winkel, G., & Redd, W. (2001). Social support, intrusive thoughts, and quality of life in breast cancer survivors. *Journal of Behavioral Medicine, 24*, 231–45.

Lickley, L. (1997). Primary breast cancer in the elderly. *Canadian Journal of Surgery, 40*, 341–51.

Macleod, U., Ross, S., Gillis, C., McConnachie, A., Twelves, C., & Watt, C. (2000). Socio-economic deprivation and stage of disease at presentation in women with breast cancer. *Annals of Oncology, 11*, 105–7.

Marrett, L.D., & Chaudhry, M. (2003). Cancer incidence and mortality in Ontario First Nations, 1968–1991 (Canada). *Cancer Causes Control, 14*, 259–68.

PART ONE

Research Design in Participatory Approaches

1 Getting Started in Research with Marginalized Populations

SUE KELLER-OLAMAN AND STEPHANIE AUSTIN

In this chapter, we focus on some of the methodological issues involved when getting participatory research projects underway. We start by building an understanding of qualitative and participatory approaches in health research and then look more closely at the methods we can apply in breast cancer settings. We discuss how to go about crafting a research question, designing a research project, recruiting participants, and gathering data – all in particular with diverse populations. To show how the practicalities of the various stages may unfold over the course of a research project, we consider case examples from Ontario Breast Cancer Community Research Initiative (OBCCRI) studies.

We also discuss how participatory breast cancer research is affected by values in the same way that health and illness are value-laden. We acknowledge that the stance we take, our research lens, and what we write are influenced by our knowledge, ideas, experiences, and the societies in which we live. What we include in this chapter is what *we* think is important to take into account when conducting research with marginalized groups of women living with breast cancer. We encourage readers to be aware of this and to ask critical questions (noting that some of the other chapters provide a more detailed description of such considerations).

Conceptual Issues

Before we discuss the design of participatory projects, we need to take a step back and touch on several underlying philosophies. Because OBCCRI projects often involve mixed methods, we briefly discuss quantitative, qualitative, and participatory approaches to research.

Quantitative and Qualitative

The quantitative approach to research is grounded in positivist and empiricist epistemologies (Creswell, 2003; Neuman, 2006). It has been the prominent theoretical perspective in mainstream science disciplines since the mid-1900s (Denzin & Lincoln, 1994). Based in the natural sciences, there are two key assumptions arising out of this philosophical approach. The first is that 'reality' is independent of and external to the observer. The second is that knowledge comes from observing or measuring this external reality. Or, simply put, 'seeing is believing.' Further assumptions include the notion that nature is orderly, and that all natural phenomena are knowable (Curtis & Taket, 1996). The positivist philosophy is reflected in the methods of quantitative studies that are based on the collection and analysis of numerical information. The focus is on seeking testable hypotheses, accurately measuring and recording the phenomena under investigation, and looking for statistical regularities or associations. Typically, large random samples are employed so the findings can be generalized to wider populations (Neuman, 2006). Quantitative research is used extensively in the study of cancer, for example, in randomized clinical drug trials or research exploring the determinants of cancer and the relationships between incidence and geography (e.g., Burris et al., 1997; Walter, Marrett, Taylor, & King, 1999).

Criticism of the quantitative approach points out that its methods do not fully account for the social and political context of the phenomenon being studied – we do not live in a laboratory setting where all external variables, other than those under investigation, can be controlled. Qualitative approaches, on the other hand, have their history in the social sciences and give greater weight to the meaning behind personal and collective experiences (Alvesson & Skoldberg, 2000; Creswell, 2003). Because individual experience is recognized as a valid way of knowing, the views of lay people are as important as the views of experts in the field (Denzin & Lincoln, 1994; Lincoln & Guba, 1985; Whitmore, 2002). This means that if we want to learn about how women with a breast cancer diagnosis cope with daily living, or what they believe is important for their health and well-being, our questions are more suited to using a qualitative approach because we are seeking to understand particular beliefs, experiences, values, and actions, rather than trying to measure and generalize the phenomenon to a broader population (Gatrell, 2002; Morse, Swanson, & Kuzel, 2001). The ultimate goal is empathetic understanding and explanation rooted in the social world rather than the natural world (Carr, 1994; Nagy Hesse-Biber & Leavy, 2003).

Qualitative research methods range from focus-group discussions and individual interviews to observations, case studies, and the analysis of documents (Denzin & Lincoln, 1994; Lincoln & Guba, 1985). Qualitative researchers also use different methods for analysing interviews and text, such as grounded theory, content analysis, and narrative analysis (Chambon, 1994; Chouliaraki & Fairclough, 2004; Krueger & Casey, 2000; Lieblich, Tuval-Mashiach, & Zilber, 1998; Parker, 2004; Rubin & Rubin, 1995). Compared to quantitative work, in qualitative work the sample – the people who will participate in the study – is usually a well-defined but small group of people. The focus is typically one of discovery and theory-generation rather than theory-testing (e.g., Barnes, Baxter, Litva, & Staples, 2002). Debates exist as to the validity of qualitative versus quantitative research (Corner, 1991). Some suggest that quantitative research using rigorous scientific research methods is the only way to obtain objective findings. That to establish causality, experiments need to be designed in such a way as to isolate the variables under investigation. And, that statistical methods must be used to ensure reliably and validity of the research results so that relationships observed between variables may be generalized to the whole population (Neuman, 2006). Others say that while the internal validity may be very high in research that uses quantitative methods, the external validity (i.e., whether the research accurately reflects real-world experiences) is weak when compared to qualitative. Qualitative researchers acknowledge, to a greater degree than their colleagues in quantitative research, how their own personal experiences are part of the research process (Morse et al., 2001). The questions asked, the interpretation of the findings, and the voices that are heard are influenced by our own values and beliefs about the world (Nagy Hesse-Biber & Leavy, 2003). We expand on the implications of this later in the chapter.

There are many different research styles that tend towards either a quantitative or qualitative paradigm. While we have described some of the quantitative and qualitative differences, we would also like to point out that there is no simple relationship between philosophical stance and methodology. There are multiple interpretations and different explanations of health and illness. Since positivists emphasize objectivity and what can be measured, they may be less likely to think of using qualitative methods. Qualitative methods are, however, used by a range of researchers and they have been employed alongside, or in conjunction with, quantitative methods (Creswell, 2003; Casebeer & Verhoef, 1997; Neuman, 2006). The two perspectives are not necessarily at odds with one another. Sometimes, mixing qualitative and quantitative approaches may be the most useful methodological strategy (see Pope & Mays, 1995). Using mixed methods can be an effective means of answering questions about the breadth of a phenomenon, as well as its depth, as opposed to just focusing on one or the other. Many OBCCRI projects involve mixed methods. Our message here is that the particular approach and chosen method will depend very much on the specific research questions to be answered. For a more detailed discussion of quantitative and qualitative differences, see Denzin and Lincoln (1994) or Pope and Mays (1995).

Participatory Research

Participatory research is a specific type of collaborative research that draws upon multiple methods, some qualitative and some quantitative (Maguire, 1987; Reitsma-Street & Brown, 2004; Ristock & Pennell, 1996). Participatory research emerged in the 1970s as an approach that would empower oppressed groups living in developing countries (Gray, Fitch, Davis, & Phillips, 2000; Kirby, Greaves, & Reid, 2006; Ristock & Pennell, 1996). A distinguishing feature is that the research participants or communities who are affected by the issues being examined engage with the researcher(s) in most phases of the project (Green et al., 1995; Reitsma-Street & Brown, 2004; St. Denis, 2004). Participants and researchers collaborate in identifying the information needed, determining the research design, collecting and analysing the data, and disseminating the results of the research (Minkler & Wallerstein, 2005).

A related key distinction of participatory approaches is that control over the research process is shared among those who are participating in the study and the researcher (Cornwall & Jewkes, 1995; Maguire, 1987; Moosa-Mitha, 2005). Unlike traditional studies, which have been criticized for being detached from the communities under study, participatory research has the ability to empower participants, as they are viewed as partners in the research process (Leung, Yen, & Minkler, 2004; Kirby et al., 2006). Activities such as sharing control in decision-making, being able to identify areas for change, and legitimizing knowledge generated by the participants all contribute to shifting the power from the researcher to the community. As communities become involved in participatory research, especially those who are marginalized by poverty, racism, or other forms of social inequality, their influence over the research process and their ability to benefit from the research outcomes can be very empowering. Participants generate knowledge about issues that directly affect them, and they engage in research that promotes change in their communities (Ristock & Pennell, 1996).

At the heart of participatory research is the notion that the end result involves the use of knowledge to take action to transform current social conditions (Hagey, 2002). The action may come in many forms and depends on the questions being asked and the community and participants who have been involved. Some examples of such action are advocacy work or disseminating the findings to those who can bring about social change. A key benefit of participatory research is that the marginalized groups involved in the research gain skills to better understand their own problems. As a result, any solutions that are developed are more relevant and accessible to the group's needs and interests than conventional research designed and undertaken at a distance from the affected communities (Gray et al., 2000; Hagey, 2002; Minkler & Wallerstein, 2005).

Participatory action research (PAR) has a very similar approach to participatory research but there is a more pronounced emphasis on action. With PAR, the goal is to develop action-based responses to problems identified by the communities or participants. For example, a PAR project may involve devising means of reducing barriers to cancer screening for women living in rural areas. All aspects of the research are action-oriented, from problem definition to research design and data collection, to analysis and dissemination of findings. PAR focuses on practical knowledge that is useful and accessible (Minkler & Wallerstein, 2005). For a more detailed discussion of PAR, see Whyte (1991) and Park, Brydon-Miller, Hall, and Jackson (1993).

To sum up, participatory research and PAR do not have distinct methods, but their unique features set them apart from more traditional research approaches. Their approaches are especially suited to work with marginalized groups because the research process exposes and challenges long-standing social and historical conditions of inequality. What this means in health settings is that the goal of the research itself is to improve the health and well-being of the participants by working to transform social forces that underlie health disparities (Cornwall & Jewkes, 1995; Gray et al., 2000).

A participatory approach in health research:

- Recognizes the social determinants of health (i.e., the importance of social, political, cultural, and economic systems in shaping health experiences, behaviours, and outcomes).
- Involves the people in the community, who share control of the entire research process.
- Emphasizes the translation of the research findings to promote changes in practice and policy.
- Is open to the use of qualitative and quantitative methods.
- Has the research goal of improving the lives of those involved (modified from Hagey, 2002).

How then, do we go about designing a participatory project with women affected by breast cancer? In the following sections, we discuss the early stages of the research project, from deciding on the topic area to recruiting participants and collecting data. Where possible, we provide examples from OBCCRI studies to show how the research process, challenges, and participatory aspects can unfold. OBCCRI projects often involve interdisciplinary and community-based research teams; they sometimes rely on mixed methods, and they always work collaboratively, drawing on health professional expertise when appropriate but focusing most on the expertise of women living with breast cancer. Although OBCCRI typically works with marginalized groups of women using participatory methods, not all projects use this approach.

Getting Started: Who and What Is Involved?

If a project is adhering to the principles of participatory research, as we have noted above, members of the community who are affected by the research being conducted will be involved at the very beginning. This could take the form of a research advisory committee or a community research team whose roles will be defined by the members of the group in the early stages of the project. In my case (SA), the project on Francophone women's experiences of breast cancer (see table 1, page 23) seemed well suited to an advisory committee formed of Francophone or Francophile women who were breast cancer survivors, service providers, and/or community workers. We met regularly over the course of the project to discuss the need for research on the experiences of

Table 1

FRANCOPHONE WOMEN WITH BREAST CANCER

Why was the research completed?
Research has shown that Francophone minorities in Ontario experience barriers in accessing health services in French, despite the Official
Languages Act in Canada, and the French Language Services Act in
Ontario. Older Francophone women in Ontario are more likely to live in
rural and remote communities, to be living on low income, and to have
lower levels of education – all of which are important determinants of
health. This project was undertaken in order to better understand the
psychosocial needs of Francophone women living with breast cancer in
Ontario.

What methods were used?
Francophone women were recruited through breast cancer organizations, health centres, and Francophone community networks. Interviews
were conducted with seven Francophone women and six cancer care
professionals in Ottawa, Toronto, and Sudbury. The interview material
was transcribed verbatim and analysed using content analysis.

What were the key findings?
Francophone women with breast cancer in Ontario have limited access
to French-language support and information, as well as to French-
speaking health professionals. The women felt that being able to speak
to professionals and support workers in their first language would have
helped them to fully understand and better cope with their illness. Only
rarely were they referred to the few existing French language sources of
information and support in Ontario.
   Results from interviews with health professionals revealed that individual efforts alone could not resolve the inequities in health services
offered to Francophone minorities in Ontario. Institutional structures
such as hospital policies and practice guidelines that support French-
language service provision in Ontario were identified as essential
mechanisms for promoting and ensuring quality cancer care in French
in Ontario.

What are some implications or results of the research?
The research contributed to raising awareness of the psychosocial
needs of Francophone women living with breast cancer in Ontario. Not

only were research results shared through presentations and publications, but the media were used to share results with the broader public.
Another concrete initiative that was undertaken following the research
was the establishment of a Francophone support group at the Centre
Francophone de Toronto. A booklet of the key findings of the study with
a list of Francophone resources that could be helpful both to health
professionals and to women living with breast cancer was developed
and distributed widely in Ontario and made available on the website of
the Centre for Research in Women's Health (http://www.crwh.org/PDF/
francophone.pdf).

Francophone women in Ontario, what the research questions would
be, who would be interviewed, and what actions could be taken with
the results of the research. Getting to know one another and building
trusting relationships was a very important part of the research process. Hearing about one another's experiences doing advocacy work on
behalf of Francophone women or providing health or information services to Francophone women was helpful in determining the gaps that
exist in support and information for this group of women living with
cancer. Also, listening to one another tell personal stories about having
had limited access to support or information in French at the time of diagnosis, treatment, or follow-up care gave the group the motivation to
conduct research that had the potential to help enhance these services
for Francophone women in Ontario.

In participatory research projects, attempts are made by researchers
and participants together to agree on a research topic, the rationale for
this particular project, the research questions, and the methods to be
used. Part of the process is also to determine what the skills are that
the participants will be building through their involvement with the
project. Community involvement can be difficult at times, and also
very rewarding. Setting the tone for fruitful collaborative relations
is crucial. Choosing members of an advisory group or a community
research team who will work well together is essential in the initial
stages of the project. Some participants or researchers may have their
own agendas that are far removed from the group's negotiated set of
agreements on what will be undertaken over the course of the research
project. Despite some of the challenges of managing group dynamics,
most would say that having a group to discuss ideas with can really

help keep the research project focused on what really matters to the community and what issues can truly be resolved through the project. Debate and difference among members of advisory groups or research teams can be very useful and insightful when they are facilitated effectively and when the members of the group are committed to working respectfully through the tensions that will inevitably come up. Making some of the possible challenges of participatory research explicit early on is one way of preventing later conflict within the group. Some participants, especially those who are living with breast cancer, may have little time and energy to devote to the project, while others may see the project as an extremely important part of their healing process and may invest considerable time and energy to this work. Given the potential constraints on a participatory process, having terms of reference for the advisory group or research team members is a good way to define in advance what expectations the group members have of one another, and how the group will work together to make decisions and move forward in their collaborative efforts.

Designing a Research Project and Crafting the Research Questions

The group's first task will be to arrive at a research topic that is meaningful to them and to others, and that is reasonable to undertake given the resources they have (e.g., time, money, willingness or capacity to be involved, access to certain communities). Sometimes, given financial and time constraints, only a small pilot project can be implemented. In a new area of research, this could be the best way to see if there is a need for this work and if there is the support and capacity for a larger study. For example, a pilot project to explore the role of the natural environment in the recovery from breast cancer treatment could be a first step in incrementally building a research program in the more general area of environment and health.

To generate discussion and ideas about participatory research, the following questions, adapted by OBCCRI researcher Chris Sinding, can help arrive at a topic:

- What are we curious about?
- What do we need to know more about?
- Are we starting from the experiences of the community?
- Do some issues need to be prioritized?
- Who will benefit from this research?

Qualitative questions can take many different forms. The list below gives an idea of the range of questions that can be asked and answered through qualitative research. In contrast to quantitative research, which asks and answers 'what' and 'where' questions at a broad population level, qualitative questions typically ask 'how' and 'why' questions at an individual or small community level.

Exploratory research questions attempt to develop a 'map of the territory' of an experience or phenomenon, for example:

• What are the key features of the breast cancer experience for older women? What 'matters' to older women about breast cancer?

Phenomenological research questions attempt to describe the essence of a phenomenon, for example:

• What is the 'essence' of caring nurse-patient interactions? What does it mean for a nurse to be 'caring' from the patients' perspectives?

Grounded theory questions attempt to reveal the process at play in a phenomenon and to build a theory, for example:

• How do women cope with a breast cancer recurrence?
• How do interactions with social workers shape the experiences of women who have a breast cancer recurrence?

Narrative research questions attempt to understand the life meaning given to events by individuals, for example:

• What is the meaning given to a breast cancer diagnosis, in the life of a young woman?

Case study questions attempt to provide an in-depth analysis of a single case, for example:

• What changes occurred in breast cancer care when Sunnybrook Health Sciences Centre and Women's College Hospital integrated and then separated?

When research design and research questions have been contemplated in general, the group must then spend time establishing exactly what they want to ask. This helps to break the topic area into more easily managed pieces, which enables the research group to be less overwhelmed and to have a clearer focus of what they are trying to achieve.

With participatory research, the community often already has some questions formulated. This was the case for me (SK) when I was approached by email and asked to evaluate 'Cottage Dreams,' a unique cancer recovery initiative (see table 2, page 28). In this program, survivors stay with family/friends or supporters for up to one week in a donated cottage. I jumped at the opportunity to be involved. As researchers, our minds are not blank slates when it comes to conducting a project. Our training, our own beliefs and feelings about the world, and the values we hold influence the topics we seek to explore, the kind of knowledge we seek to generate, the questions we ask, and the way we go about actually doing the research through to the end. I started with an interest in the work and some assumptions about the value of the Cottage Dreams experience for women with breast cancer. I was not pushing for the results to emerge a certain way, but I believe that this is an important area and I do carry the assumption that spending time in natural environments can have a healing effect for many people. I also believe that the more we learn about the relationships among environments and quality of life and health the better we will be able to help improve the lives of women affected by breast cancer.

Cottage Dreams: More Than a Vacation

Following several emails, phone calls, and one in-person meeting, I agreed to undertake the evaluation of the Cottage Dreams program and provide regular updates to the advisory group. The advisory group was composed of the Cottage Dreams president, a clinical practitioner/academic, and a research consultant. Hagey (2002) describes this type of work as evaluative participatory action research; it draws from participatory action research traditions but the purpose and design are clearly focused on evaluation. The group would share their expertise and hands-on experience and provide feedback to guide the evaluation. The project called for some quantitative but mainly qualitative methods. The quantitative component involved summarizing records of how many people had applied and been placed in a cottage – data that had been collected over several years. The qualitative piece involved reading the feedback comment sheets and conducting indi-

Table 2

COTTAGE DREAMS

Why was the research completed?
Cottage Dreams is a unique recovery initiative offered to people that
have completed cancer treatment in the past nine months. Survivors
stay with family, friends, or supporters for one week in a donated cottage, often in spectacular natural settings. The program, established in
2003, was very well received but had not been formally evaluated.

   This project was conducted to help Cottage Dreams understand what
the program means to recipients and to gather suggestions for future
directions. In addition, the project provided the opportunity to explore the
wider question about environmental issues and concerns that are important in everyday lives and about positive aspects of the environment for
those affected by cancer and recovering from treatment.

What methods were used?
An advisory group guided the work. First, the number of cottage
placements each year was summarized quantitatively, using data that
was already collected by Cottage Dreams. Second, thirty-five written
feedback cards were scanned and individual qualitative interviews were
conducted with twenty-three women affected by breast cancer and with
nine supporters who had experienced the program. Interview areas
included: what they would tell others to expect from the program, the
extent to which the cottage experience is part of healing and recovery,
challenges, and suggestions for future directions.

What were the key findings?
Recovering after cancer treatment is different for everyone, as are the
effects of cancer itself. Overall, views of the program were very positive
and included an appreciation of: a natural setting, relaxing atmosphere,
a celebration following treatment, a chance to talk and spend time with
friends/family, a chance to feel more 'normal,' and an opportunity to reflect on what had happened and bring emotional aspects to the fore. The
majority of challenges identified were minor practical issues. However,
occasionally aspects of the application process (the paperwork, the
screening interview) or perceptions of overworked staff were noted.

What are some implications or results of the research?
Cottage Dreams demonstrated the ability to positively influence the lives

of cancer survivors and their supporters. It was also encouraging that the program was receptive to new ideas. As a result of this project, Cottage Dreams has changed the application process and the information packages that are sent to recipients. This project also contributes to knowledge about characteristics of environments and 'place' that are important for women affected by breast cancer.

vidual in-depth interviews to determine the extent to which and the ways in which the cottage week influenced health, healing, and quality of life for the participants. The feedback sheets had closed and open-ended questions.

In the initial stages of the research, members of the team had different ideas for how the research should be designed and what methods should be used. The group had clear but sometimes different ideas of what they wanted to ask to get the cottage project underway. Some of the group members felt that 'before and after' surveys were needed in order to capture the impact of the cottage week. The information could then be graphed, which would produce visually appealing results that could help influence potential program sponsors. After talking among the group, however, we realized that it would not be possible due to the few cancer patients scheduled to stay in cottages over the upcoming winter months. Moreover, if we wanted to capture the experiences, thoughts, and feelings participants had in relation to Cottage Dreams, a significant part of the evaluation would need a qualitative approach. Therefore, one of the first steps involved reshaping some of the key questions. We achieved this through discussion of the program's goals, the limitations of the evaluation, and how Cottage Dreams hoped to use the research.

Drawing on the different methods, the cottage evaluation was designed to answer three key questions: 1) What does the program mean to recipients? 2) What aspects of the (physical and/or social) environment matter for health, healing, and quality of life for women affected by breast cancer? 3) How is the program part of healing and recovery?

Cottage Interviews

The women affected by breast cancer and their husbands/partners who had stayed in a Cottage Dreams donated cottage were interviewed on separate occasions. Initially the women were asked questions to gain a sense of where they see themselves at present and how they describe their health and quality of life. They were then asked about the actual program and what makes the cottage experience so special. The following interview questions were used to guide discussion with Cottage Dreams participants:

- If you were a Cottage Dreams coordinator and I was a survivor, what would you tell me to expect from this program?
- Can you talk about Cottage Dreams as part of your healing and recovery process? (whether positive or negative)
- Why do you think the cottage experience is so special – often described as 'more than a vacation'?

The final question was asked to explore features of the cottage experience that were especially important for cancer survivors. This question was posed to gain insight into what may be missing from the general environment that only a cottage experience could provide. The Cottage Dreams evaluation touched on part of the broad research area of environment and health, which aims to build knowledge about aspects of the physical and social environments that matter for women following breast cancer treatment.

Recruitment

Locating and recruiting participants in a participatory project is an essential component of the research process. Creative and innovative ideas can sometimes be very useful for reaching sub-groups of the population who may be marginalized and difficult to reach. Members of the research team or advisory group can bring information about the types of participants being recruited to their networks and help spread the word about the project. For example, with the Cottage Dreams study, recruitment was carried out by the recovery program staff. They used their database and sent emails, inviting those who had stayed in a cottage to participate. Replies from those wishing to take part were forwarded to me. This approach was successful and resulted in a response rate of 67 per cent.

Recruitment for the Cottage Dreams study was relatively straightforward and consisted of a group of women who were similar across two main variants of interest – having been part of the Cottage Dreams recovery initiative and recovering after treatment. In the breast cancer context it is important to consider selection details such as these, as well as other recruitment particulars such as age at diagnosis or 'life stage' at time of diagnosis because concerns may differ between older and younger women. In addition, aspects such as time since diagnosis (e.g., recently diagnosed versus longer-term survivors), geographic location, education level achieved, employment status, and ethnic identity may play an important role in the lived experience of women living with breast cancer and should therefore be thought through in research design – especially in determining the selection criteria for the sample of research participants and their recruitment into the study (e.g., Wright, Corner, Hopkinson, & Foster, 2006; Ziebland et al., 2004). This is linked to the concern around over-researching the same groups of women, which produces research that is less representative of the full range of women who are affected by breast cancer.

When using the focus group as a method of data collection, it can be helpful to recruit participants who have some similar experiences to ensure that focus group participants have enough common ground to feel safe sharing their experiences with strangers during a group interview. Although the intention behind focus groups as a data collection method is not to achieve consensus, some amount of common experience is essential in the design and recruitment of participants for a focus group. However, limited time and resources may require researchers to occasionally combine women with very different experiences – for example, women working as health professionals and women living as cancer survivors – within one group. It is also important to note that an over-reliance on a single strategy or source for recruitment (e.g., via emails, listservs, or through one health service provider or cancer centre) can limit the range of participants and perhaps reduce the scope and applicability of the research. For instance, recruiting research participants through health service providers exclusively may limit respondents to those women who have received services recently.

In the project on Francophone women with breast cancer, I (SA) recruited participants through existing breast cancer networks in Toronto, Sudbury, and Ottawa via community organizations and cancer centres who were known by the project's research advisory committee. I also made posters and short invitations informing potential participants of the research project and encouraging them to contact me should they be interested in this opportunity to discuss their experiences as Franιορhone women with breast cancer or as health professionals serving this population. I published this invitation in a breast cancer newsletter that is distributed widely across Ontario. I used email and print media to advertise the study, drawing attention to the unique nature of this project. It was important that there be regional, geographical, and ethnic diversity in the group that would become my sample. Furthermore, I wanted the group to include women with a range of experiences related to their age at breast cancer onset, breast cancer stage, and overall experiences with the cancer care system. In the sample of health professionals, I wanted a range of service providers working as nurses, social workers, and physicians.

Some of the challenges included accessing the full range of diverse experiences of breast cancer care in Ontario. I was unable to find a Francophone oncologist to interview and therefore had to be content with a convenience sample representing a smaller range of health professionals working in the area. Similarly, by having used written calls for participation more often than verbal ones, my sample may have been limited to participants who could read.

So far, we have outlined how to craft a research question and some elements to take into account when recruiting people for participatory projects. In the following section, we consider how to collect data. It is beyond the scope of this chapter to mention every data collection technique, but we provide an overview of a number of commonly used techniques, and then focus on a form often used in OBCCRI studies.

Gathering Data

As we mentioned earlier, participatory research is not a method but a specific orientation to research. In terms of data collection, either qualitative or quantitative methods, or a mixture of both, may be used. The chosen method(s) should best fit the nature of the phenomena being studied. There must also be agreement between the researchers and the community as to which methods will be most appropriate (Minkler & Wallerstein, 2005).

Surveys and Interviews

Both quantitative and qualitative studies may use surveys or individual interviews. In our own work, some of these techniques overlap. For example, evaluating the Cottage Dreams program (SK) called for both in-depth individual interviews to explore personal experiences and statistical analysis of existing data to describe the number of cottage placements per year. Focus groups, which may be thought of as a collective interview, are also a popular technique. The interviews and focus groups can be conducted in person or via the phone and are usually audio-taped and transcribed. The quantitative-qualitative difference, however, lies in the level of structure imposed.

With quantitative surveys and interviews, structure is important in order to control the uniformity of data collection for making predictions and generalizing to larger populations (Gatrell, 2002; Neuman, 2006). Quantitative paper and pencil questionnaires are not intended to allow for open opinions or views. Similarly, a quantitative interview follows a rigid form where the interviewer does not deviate from the wording of the questions. Examples of typical quantitative data sources include censuses and routinely recorded data (such as the cancer registry).

In contrast, qualitative data collection encourages free and open responses with the added bonus of capturing participants' perceptions in their own words (Rubin & Rubin, 1995; Whitmore, 2002). Surveys allow open-ended responses and the interview schedule is semi-structured or unstructured to allow for the exploration of responses and comments.

Focus Groups

We now devote more attention to focus groups, as this method for collecting data is common in OBCCRI projects. A focus group involves a small number of people plus a facilitator who have been brought together to discuss a particular issue (Krueger & Casey, 2000). Usually the members of a group have a common interest or share a characteristic relevant to the research (e.g., Francophone women with breast cancer). The discussions are relatively informal, with the goal of collecting an 'insider's view' and thereby producing measures with strong validity. Group dynamics also come into play with the hope that the interaction and differences of opinion amongst the group will yield more data and insight than interviews with individuals (Patton, 2001). Focus groups are most appropriate for exploring the breadth of an issue – that is, the range and scope, rather than the frequency. Focus groups are also useful when probing for information about sensitive topics, generating or introducing new ideas, or seeking targeted viewpoints.

An additional aspect to consider is the composition of the group. As noted in the recruitment section, a participant's age, education level, stage in the cancer trajectory, and so on, will all be important because they influence the dynamics between the researcher and the group. Determining how many groups are needed is another aspect, along with determining where the groups will be held and how structured the discussion is going to be. Even with a flexible topic guide, the researcher should be able to provide a clear aim and purpose of the group(s). Once the focus group data is collected, some participatory researchers feel it is important to include the participants in the data analysis and interpretation phases to ensure that the findings reflect the views of the group.

It is always advisable to know the limitations inherent in one's research design to minimize their impact, if possible, and to know how they may shape the extent and quality of the data gathered.

Reflection and Reflexivity

Why is reflection a big deal in qualitative research? The quality of the research ultimately rests on the thoughtfulness, inquisitiveness, and attentiveness of those who do the research. The researchers, along with their advisory group or research team, are designing the research, devising the research questions, collecting the data, and interpreting this material with the conceptual and analytic tools they have gained over their lifetimes. Much depends on the quality of the reflection and the reflexivity between the participants' shared ideas and experiences, and the researchers' ideas and experiences. Reflecting on our research questions raises awareness of the researchers' 'presence' in the research process. We create worlds through the questions we ask in qualitative research. When our questions are thoughtfully combined with what our research participants regard as reasonable responses, interpretive material is created. So, simply put, asking critical, thoughtful, and provocative questions of yourself, your participants, and your data in the analysis stage will deeply affect the results of the research.

In addition to the interpretive lens of the research participant, which is called upon during the interview, the researcher's interpretation is actively engaged in the research process – at the design stage, in the interview exchange, as well as during the analysis and writing stages. Furthermore, in the design of our studies, participants are involved not only in the interview, but also at a later stage in the research process when we invite them to reinterpret our accounts of their life experiences. This thorough interpretive practice makes possible the richness of description that can be found in participatory research that uses qualitative methods.

Methodological Challenges – Practical and Personal

Participatory research accents partnerships, capacity building, shared expertise, learning, and a push for social change. However, in reality, participatory research does not always flow smoothly. What does participation actually mean? There are varying levels of involvement – sometimes the participants do not want a great deal of control over the research process. Enthusiasm for projects ebbs and flows – while the participants may have energy and ideas to start with, we have seen enthusiasm decline, especially when an individual's ideas do not end up being incorporated in the project.

There is also the position in which the researcher may find herself. Researchers should be careful in their use of 'participatory' so that it does not become a token term for simply involving participants in any research (Gray et al., 2000). It is also important to rouse interest in the community, while not giving false hope. Having said this, discussing what the project can and can not do early on is an important reality check (Cornwall & Jewkes, 1995). Participatory research aims to work with the participants or community. Often it is assumed that those involved are a relatively homogeneous group, and we often try to achieve this via our recruiting for focus groups. As you will see in OBCCRI work, however (e.g., in the Francophone women study), this is often a simplification. Group members may have strong networks, but they vary across age, religion, income level, and views of priorities.

Another participatory research challenge lies in time considerations. A participatory approach requires commitment and time from those involved. Although the community may be very keen to partner in the research, in our experience, many of the groups we reach are made up of volunteers who have demanding workloads. They have too little time to be as involved as they may wish. Another issue to be aware of when deciding on a data collection method is who is going to collect the data. If it is going to be those in the community, training may be needed and the process may take longer. In addition, if the researcher is a student with certain research deadlines, there is not a great deal of flexibility for those who need more time because they have deviated from their original proposal – a turn which can happen due to the adaptable nature of participatory work, Leung et al. (2004) go so far as to suggest that this style of research not be carried out if the timeline does not allow education and action as part of the process. We would add that the publication of findings is another time-related factor. Ideally the dissemination strategy should be discussed in advance. From our experience, the dissemination of the findings is left to the researcher, with occasional input from the community partners.

Funding is also an issue. Community groups are often at a disadvantage when it comes to understanding the procedures and eligibility criteria of a research funding organization (Gray et al., 2000). Due to a lack of experience with research and with funding applications, community groups may not be able to participate as equal partners in this part of the process. It is also expensive to conduct interviews and focus groups, especially when travel is involved.

Despite the challenges, the participatory research experience can provide plenty of benefits when a good partnership is established, advancing knowledge, mutual learning, and, most importantly, the health and well-being of marginalized groups. Part of the commitment to participatory work also involves being able to walk away or disengage from a project if any of the contributing parties are no longer able to deliver on the commitments made. Walking away may also be linked to questions about the ownership of the information or an examination of one's values and beliefs. The beliefs and attitudes of the researcher are an important part of participatory research which stimulates critical thought and questions the role of the researcher.

Conclusion

This chapter has focused on participatory research, which offers a different approach to collecting and analysing data than do more traditional research methods. Participatory research facilitates capacity building in the community, mutual learning, and knowledge production and exchange. Yet, there are many questions to think about before getting a project underway. This chapter has also highlighted methodological issues of participatory research and illustrated that high quality research and community involvement are not contrary to each other. This chapter also posed some questions and challenges – not least of which is the challenge to the researchers themselves. There is a special attitude; where experiential knowledge is valued, knowledge is democratized, and power is shared throughout the research process. And ultimately, in true participatory research, the ownership of the data sits with the participants or community partners (Leung et al., 2004). In terms of the methods we have described or presented, we are not offering a prescription to follow as one size does not fit all. One needs to select the methods appropriate to the research question and data available – and enjoy the work and wealth of learning that comes with this approach.

Acknowledgments

FRANCOPHONE WOMEN WITH BREAST CANCER STUDY
Principal Investigator: Stephanie Austin
Advisory Group Members: Lucie Chauvette, Anemia Institute; Carol Burnham Cook, Willow Breast Cancer Support and Resource Services; Claire Parrot, Rouge Valley Health Systems; Simone Durantet, Centre medico-social communautaire; Manon Labrecque, Ontario Breast Cancer Community Research Initiative.

This project was funded by the Ontario Breast Cancer Community Research Initiative, which is funded by the Canadian Breast Cancer Foundation, Ontario Chapter.

COTTAGE DREAMS STUDY
Principal Investigator: Sue Keller-Olaman
Advisory Group Members: Seana O'Neill, Susan Lenard, Dr. Claire Crooks

We would also like to thank all of the women who participated in the project.

This project was funded by the Ontario Breast Cancer Community Research Initiative, which is funded by the Canadian Breast Cancer Foundation, Ontario Chapter.

REFERENCES

Alvesson, M., & Skoldberg, K. (2000). *Reflexive methodology: New vistas for qualitative research.* London: Sage.
Barnes, G., Baxter, J., Litva, A., & Staples, B. (2002). The social and psychological impact of the chemical contamination incident in Weston Village, UK: A qualitative analysis. *Social Science and Medicine, 55,* 2227–41.
Burris, H., Moore, M., Andersen, J., Green, M., Rothenberg, M., Modiano, M.,

et al. (1997). Improvements in survival and clinical benefit with gemcitabine as first-line therapy for patients with advanced pancreas cancer: A randomized trial. *Journal of Clinical Oncology, 15*(6), 2403–13.

Carr, L. (1994). The strengths and weaknesses of quantitative and qualitative research: What method for nursing? *Journal of Advanced Nursing, 20*, 716–21.

Casebeer, A., & Verhoef, M. (1997). Combining qualitative and quantitative research methods: Considering the possibilities for enhancing the study of chronic diseases. *Chronic Diseases in Canada, 18*(3), 130–5.

Chambon, A. (1994). The dialogical analysis of case materials. In E. Sherman & W. Reid (Eds.), *Qualitative research in social work* (pp. 205–15). New York: Columbia University Press.

Chouliaraki, L., & Fairclough, N. (2004). The critical analysis of discourse. In W. Carroll (Ed.), *Critical strategies for social research* (pp. 262–75). Toronto, ON: Canadian Scholars' Press.

Corner, J. (1991). In search of more complete answers to research questions. Quantitative versus qualitative research methods: Is there a way forward? *Journal of Advanced Nursing, 16*(6), 718–27.

Cornwall, A., & Jewkes, R. (1995). What is participatory research? *Social Science and Medicine, 41*(12), 1667–76.

Creswell, J. (2003). *Research design: Qualitative, quantitative and mixed method approaches* (2nd ed.). Thousand Oaks, CA: Sage.

Curtis, S., & Taket, A. (1996). Changing perspectives on health and societies. In S. Curtis, A. Taket, & A.R. Taket (Eds.), *Health and society: Changing perspectives*. New York: John Wiley & Sons.

Denzin, N., & Lincoln, Y. (1994). *Handbook of qualitative research*. Thousand Oaks, CA: Sage.

Gatrell, A. (2002). Explaining geographies of health. In A. Gatrell (Ed.), *Geographies of health: An introduction*. Oxford: Blackwell Publishers.

Gray, R., Fitch, M., Davis, C., & Phillips, C. (2000). Challenges of participatory research: Reflections on a study with breast cancer self-help groups. *Health Expectations, 3*, 243–52.

Green, L., George, M., Daniel, M., Frankish, C., Herbert, C., Bowie, W., et al. (1995). *Study of participatory research in health promotion: Review and recommendations for the development of participatory research in health promotion in Canada*. Ottawa: Royal Society of Canada.

Hagley, R. (2002). Guest editorial: The use and abuse of participatory research. Retrieved March 2006 from http://www.phac-aspc.gc.ca/publicat/cdic-mcc/18-1/a_e.html

Kirby, S., Greaves, L., & Reid, C. (2006). *Experience, research, social change: Methods beyond the mainstream*. Toronto, ON: Broadview Press.

Krueger, R., & Casey, M. (2000). *Focus groups: A practical guide for applied research* (3rd ed.). Newbury Park, CA: Sage.

Leung, M., Yen, I., & Minkler, M. (2004). Community-based participatory research: A promising approach for increasing epidemiology's relevance in the 21st century. *International Journal of Epidemiology, 33*, 499–506.

Lieblich, A., Tuval-Mashiach, R., & Zilber, T. (1998). *Narrative research: Reading, analysis, and interpretation.* Thousand Oaks, CA: Sage.

Lincoln, Y., & Guba, E. (1985). *Naturalistic inquiry.* Beverly Hills, CA: Sage.

Maguire, P. (1987). *Doing participatory research: A feminist approach.* Amherst, MA: Center for International Education.

Minkler, M., & Wallerstein, N. (2005). *Community-based participatory research for health* (2nd ed.). San Francisco, CA: Jossey-Bass.

Moosa-Mitha, M. (2005). Situating anti-oppressive theories within critical and difference-centred perspectives. In I. Brown & S. Strega (Eds.), *Research as resistance: Critical, indigenous, and anti-oppressive approaches* (pp. 237–54). Toronto, ON: Canadian Scholars' Press.

Morse, J., Swanson, J., & Kuzel, A. (Eds.). (2001). *The nature of qualitative evidence.* Thousand Oaks, CA: Sage.

Nagy Hesse-Biber, S., & Leavy, P. (Eds.). (2003). *Approaches to qualitative research: A reader on theory and practice.* Oxford: Oxford University Press.

Neuman, L. (2006). *Social research methods: Qualitative and quantitative approaches* (6th ed.). Boston: Allyn & Bacon.

Park, P., Brydon-Miller, M., Hall, B., & Jackson, T. (Eds.). (1993). *Voices of change: Participatory research in the United States and Canada.* Westport, CT: Bergin & Garvey.

Parker, I. (2004). Discovering discourses, tackling texts. In W. Carroll (Ed.), *Critical strategies for social research.* Toronto, ON: Canadian Scholars' Press.

Patton, M. (2001). *Qualitative evaluation and research methods* (3rd ed.). Newbury Park, CA: Sage.

Pope, C., & Mays, N. (1995). Qualitative research: Reaching the parts other methods cannot reach: An introduction to qualitative methods in health and health services research. *British Medical Journal, 311*, 42–5.

Reitsma-Street, M., & Brown, L. (2004). Community action research. In W. Carroll (Ed.), *Critical strategies for social research* (pp. 303–19). Toronto, ON: Canadian Scholars' Press.

Ristock, J., & Pennell, J. (1996). *Community research as empowerment: Feminist links, postmodern interruptions.* Toronto: Oxford University Press.

Rubin, H., & Rubin, I. (1995). *Qualitative interviewing: The art of hearing data.* Thousand Oaks, CA: Sage.

St. Denis, V. (2004). Community-based participatory research: Aspects of the

40   Cancer on the Margins

concept relevant for practice, In W. Carroll (Ed.), *Critical strategies for social research* (pp. 292–302). Toronto, ON: Canadian Scholars' Press.

Walter, S., Marrett, L., Taylor, S.M., & King, D. (1999). An analysis of the geographic variation in cancer incidence and its determinants in Ontario. *Canadian Journal of Public Health, 90*(2), 104–8.

Whitmore, E. (2002). They listened to what we had to say: Emancipatory evaluation. In I. Shaw & N. Gould (Eds.), *Qualitative inquiry* (pp. 79–91). Thousand Oaks, CA: Wadsworth.

Whyte, W. (1991). *Participatory action research*. Newbury Park, CA: Sage.

Wright, D., Corner, J., Hopkinson, J., & Foster, C. (2006). Listening to the views of people affected by cancer about cancer research: An example of participatory research in setting the cancer research agenda. *Health Expectations, 9*, 3–12.

Ziebland, S., Chapple, A., Dumelow, C., Evans, J., Prinjha, S., & Rozmovits, L. (2004). How the Internet affects patients' experience of cancer: A qualitative study. *British Medical Journal, 328*, 564–70.

2 Ethical Considerations in Participatory Breast Cancer Research

STEPHANIE AUSTIN

Conducting participatory research on women's experiences of breast cancer involves collaboration among differentially positioned individuals – researchers, health professionals, community groups, and concerned citizens. Each stakeholder group represents a constituency that has ethical codes of conduct to guide its research activities. This chapter will discuss the processes involved in negotiating academic and community needs and expectations in an effort to engage in ethical research. The broad social and political landscape of breast cancer research will be critically analysed to determine whose needs are being served by the research (e.g., funders, academics, organizations, consumer groups, individual patients). I will address the tensions and ethical dilemmas involved in ensuring that the needs of marginalized social groups are being met. Case examples from my work will draw attention to the ethical implications of working across differences in participatory breast cancer research.

The Broader Context: Working Ethically

In Canada, the Social Sciences and Humanities Research Council (SSHRC), the Canadian Institutes of Health Research (CIHR), and the Natural Sciences and Engineering Research Council (NSERC), known as the Tri-council, have developed ethical guidelines to ensure minimum harm and maximum benefit in research. The ethical principles guiding research activity in Canada are the following: respect for human dignity, respect for free and informed consent, respect for vulnerable persons, respect for privacy and confidentiality, respect for justice and inclusiveness, balancing harms and benefits, minimizing harms, maximizing benefits (Canada, 2003). Ethical review has become a requirement of most research granting agencies, universities, and academic hospitals in Canada.

For each research project, researchers need to write an ethical protocol and submit it to an ethical review board. These boards are often located in hospitals or universities. They are composed of researchers, some of whom may have particular expertise in research ethics. Community members or patients sometimes participate in ethical review boards as well. The general principles and processes guiding ethical research in Canada translate into common practices and procedures when conducting participatory research. The focus here will be on how principles of respect for justice and inclusiveness, for example, manifest in the day to day work of those engaged in participatory research.

There are some common ethical problems in participatory research. For instance, quite often, research is not directly relevant to the communities for whom the research is intended. Communities who participate in research may experience or perceive coercion or manipulation through the research process, and may not have access to the benefits of the research. As a result, many communities feel over-researched or experience 'research fatigue.'

Research questions tend to be framed from the perspective of the researcher, who is often less focused than community groups on questions like 'what shall we do about it?' For example, in cancer research contexts, researchers may be concerned with why cancer is so prevalent in one community compared to another, or why services are available for this community and not that community, but they may not have the training, resources, or inclination to follow those questions up with strategies to implement and evaluate changes to the fundamental problems that are identified through the research. Another common ethical problem arises when resources are spent on research in cases where solutions to community problems exist that are simpler and more cost-effective than those being researched. Ethical codes that take community voices into account are of critical importance in resolving these problems. Aboriginal groups have taken a leadership role in developing such community-based ethical research guidelines.

Some may suggest that common sense could help us avoid some of these pitfalls. Often this is true. We all have personal ethical codes of conduct that guide our actions. However, ethical review boards have been put in place to ensure that researchers or research projects do not do unintentional harm. The ethical review process requires that we consider ethical issues 'up front.' This process provides ample opportunity for the research team to discuss issues and come up with potential solutions in advance. It forces researchers to put on paper how they will handle potential ethical conflicts, and allows for the identification of problems before they happen. It also ensures that 'objective' or more distanced observers review the research process.

According to community researchers Rosa, Russell, and Prilleltensky (1996), every aspect of research involves choice points in which we can decide to promote equity or not. These choices are guided by ethics. Historically, research has implicitly or explicitly been oriented towards serving the needs of dominant groups, as in the case of Aboriginal peoples. Indeed, in *Decolonizing Methodologies*, Tuhiwai Smith (1999) argues convincingly:

> The ways in which scientific research is implicated in the worst excesses of colonialism remains a powerful remembered history for many of the world's colonized peoples. It is a history that still offends the deepest sense of our humanity. Just knowing that someone measured our 'faculties' by filling the skulls of our ancestors with millet seeds and compared the amount of millet seed to the capacity for mental thought offends our sense of who and what we are. (p. 1)

The racism, sexism, classism, and other forms of oppression that have been perpetuated in the name of research are disturbing realities. Acknowledging this historical and contemporary phenomenon, we need to continually ask ourselves what kinds of alternatives can be developed. Community researchers in Canada have actively endeavoured to create research methodologies that transform inequitable power imbalances and ensure that the benefits of research are shared equitably among research partners (Kirby, Greaves, & Reid, 2006). Ristock and Pennell (1996) advance the notion that empowerment as a goal of community research implies consciously thinking about gendered, racialized, and other relations of power to enhance critical analysis throughout the research process (see also Reitsma-Street & Brown, 2004; St. Denis, 2004). This is the orientation I brought to my research with a marginalized group of women living with breast cancer.

Setting the Stage: Working Collaboratively

Building partnerships and relationships is a central feature of designing and conducting ethical participatory research (Muzychka & Poulin, 1995). Ensuring minimum harm and maximum benefit to communities involved in research requires an intimate knowledge of the changing needs of the communities with whom we are working. This knowledge is acquired through reciprocal dialogue. Relationships of trust take time to develop, especially with groups who have been marginalized by socioeconomic oppression, racism, or homophobia (Carroll, 2004).

My experience conducting a pilot study on the information and support needs of Francophone women living with breast cancer in Ontario (see table 1, page 23) involved attempts to establish working relationships within a very short time frame. Working collaboratively with marginalized communities, like Francophones in Ontario, who are scattered across the province and represent only 5 per cent of the Ontario population as a whole, tends to require more time and more resources for communication, coordination, and travel. As a Franco-Ontarian woman myself, I was aware of some of the social, political, and economic inequalities that place this social group at the margins. Their access to health and social services in their language is especially compromised. I was aware of the importance and value of aligning myself, and this study, with established and trustworthy community organizations and healthcare facilities that had a history of meeting the health and social needs of minority Francophones. In light of common constraints, I was committed to working collaboratively – sharing ideas, resources, networks, and outcomes of the research.

My desire to work with a community health centre (CHC) whose mandate was to serve minority Francophones in Toronto did not always fit within this CHC's workload, which was already full to capacity. While research on the particular needs of Francophone women living with breast cancer was somewhat related to the health centre's mandate, and could eventually be helpful in their work, the centre had many other priorities that needed immediate attention.

It would have taken years of trust-building to develop a common agenda and streamline a process of approval and effective decision-making between my academic institution and their community organization. I met several times with the director of this organization, and with the clinical and community development staff. In principle, they were eager to support this work. In practice, our working relationships were tentative and ultimately followed parallel tracks. More concretely, the project never made it onto the agenda of the monthly board of directors meetings of this CHC during the course of the project. However, the organization did promote the project by contributing to spreading the word about the study in their waiting room, newsletter, and by word of mouth. They also participated in disseminating the results of the study once it was completed.

I also attempted to build effective partnerships with health professionals who worked with linguistic minorities in Ontario, especially social workers, nurses, physicians, and oncologists from cancer centres in Toronto, Ottawa, and Sudbury. As is often the case when attempting to work on behalf of marginalized social groups, I was able to find one or two key allies in each cancer centre who later became links with their organizations. Working with researchers and health professionals in Ottawa and Sudbury while I was in Toronto proved challenging, even when there was an expressed desire to collaborate. Formal relationships were difficult to establish across different institutions. Because the ethical procedures were not harmonized among institutions, to fully integrate health professionals as co-researchers in the project, I would have had to submit adapted applications to fulfil the requirements of each separate ethics review board. This process could have taken the whole year within which the project needed to be completed.

Since 2004, a number of Toronto institutions have harmonized their ethical procedures. This harmonization ensures that the ten participating health centres, hospitals, and university sites have common protocols and review boards for research conducted in Toronto. Ultimately, when institutional arrangements are not harmonized, collaboration is difficult, if not impossible. This may compromise the quality of health research, and eventually of healthcare. The best research, and the best healthcare, may end up existing in places where a few committed individuals with access to resources have worked to create better systems and structures of collaboration and communication. This creates a deep ethical concern for researchers who are attempting to enhance the well-being of marginalized social groups, especially because resources are likely to be scarce or non-existent.

Ethical conflicts abound in collaborative approaches to research. There are many more acknowledged sources of personal, interpersonal, and political conflict in participatory research than in non-participatory research. Opening oneself up to the possibilities that collaborative research engenders can be exhilarating and validating, as well as risky. The process of bringing ourselves into our research practices can be uooful, and sometimes intimidating. Locating ourselves within the research, rather than remaining distanced observers, requires a level of commitment, engagement, and honesty that is difficult to sustain at times, but which is necessary when working across social differences (Moosa-Mitha, 2005). Donna Haraway suggests that 'location is about vulnerability; location resists the politics of closure, finality' and adds that a feminist approach 'resists fixation and is insatiably curious about the webs of differential positioning' (1991, p. 196). The potential for learning and change in this approach to research is immense.

Getting the Job Done – Working the System

There are several steps involved in obtaining ethical approval for research. In this section, I will present an overview of the elements that go into an application for ethical review. At each step, I will pose some critical questions and give some examples of where ethical issues can arise, and what to keep in mind when determining how to resolve them.

Purpose of the Research

The first stage of any application for ethical approval involves writing a summary of the research, which generally includes a few short paragraphs explaining the background, rationale, and objectives. Questions to help animate thinking at this stage include the following:

- Is this research really justified?
- Who will benefit from this work and how?
- How was the community involved or consulted in defining the research need?
- Who came up with the objectives and how?
- Are there concrete action outcomes in this project?

Answering these questions will help clarify and strengthen the logic or rationale to justify each step of the research process. In my study of Francophone women's information and support needs, one of the first steps was to establish an advisory committee composed of people who were directly touched by the issues. The group consisted of Francophone women who were living with breast cancer, some who were health and social service providers, and some who had been involved in advocacy. This group helped define the research needs of this community of women. They shared their experiences and expertise to validate or challenge my ideas about the purpose of the study, the potential benefits of the study, and the potential pitfalls.

Research Methods

In this section of the ethics protocol, the researcher must describe exactly how the research will be carried out. Questions related to the *who, what, when, where,* and *why* of this research project are answered in this section. The procedures used in the study are identified (e.g., interviews, questionnaires) and the time frame for the research is stated (e.g., how long each procedure will take, how long the research will last overall). Some questions to animate thinking at this next stage might include the following:

- How will the community be involved?
- What training or capacity-building opportunities will be built in?
- Will the methods used be sensitive and appropriate to various communities (e.g., considering literacy, language barriers, cultural sensitivities)?
- How will scientific rigour and accessibility be balanced?

Adapting the research methodology to the participant community is extremely important. For example, using a survey questionnaire with participants who may be illiterate can be inappropriate and ineffective. In my study with Francophone women, I chose to meet individually with each participant as a means of establishing a trusting bond that would allow for more in-depth sharing of personal experiences, such as feeling misunderstood, mistreated, or somehow alienated in an Anglophone cancer care system. Consider what one participant had to say about the difference it would have made had she been able to express herself in French:

> le sens de l'humour, la douceur des paroles, c'est à la maison, finalement, le français, alors ça, ça aurait été réconfortant ... c'est certain que ça calme d'être dans un contexte qui nous est familier, dans un contexte ou j'veux dire, tu le sais, étant bilingue, on est pas la même personne en anglais qu'on l'est en français. [the sense of humour, the gentleness of the words, it's at home, French, in the end, so that would have been comforting ... it certainly is calming to be in a familiar context, in a context where I mean,

you know, being bilingual, we're not the same person in English as we are in French.] (Translated from French as cited in Austin, 2004)

Research Participants

The next section to include in the ethics protocol is a description of the participants in the study. It is important to describe how they will be selected, explicitly stating the criteria used (e.g., age when diagnosed with cancer, stage of cancer, primary language spoken). It is also essential to discuss the proposed sample size (i.e., how many people will be involved in this study and why). Special issues concerning the proposed populations would also be described in this section. For instance, if I had been interviewing an under eighteen year old daughter of a Francophone woman with breast cancer, I would have had to obtain parental approval for this person's participation. Protecting or being conscientious of the particular needs of vulnerable groups is essential in ethical research. Some additional questions to consider:

- Who are the 'right' people to answer the research questions most appropriately (e.g., service providers, community members, leaders)?
- Will the research process engage marginalized or disenfranchised groups or individuals?
- Who speaks for the community?
- Is there a reason to exclude some people?

In qualitative research especially, researchers are not attempting to discover trends that can be generalized in the whole population; rather, we are trying to inquire into the *why* and *how* of particular lived experiences. The choice of *who* to interview is therefore of critical importance. Having clear selection criteria with a strong rationale is essential in order to justify not only the ethics of the project, but also its value throughout the research process and after its completion. Questions about who was included and who was excluded from the research will often be asked. A well-articulated logic for these choices is of utmost importance.

Recruitment

Another section required in an ethics protocol is one that describes how the participants will be recruited. It is important to remember that effective recruitment relies on many diverse mechanisms – some written and some oral – to ensure that even those with low literacy may be informed of the study. How and by whom participants will be approached and asked to participate should be stated. Copies of the recruitment materials should be included (e.g., posters, advertisements, letters). It is important to identify institutions or locations from which participants will be recruited (e.g., hospital, clinic, school) and to provide a statement of the investigator's relationship, if any, to the participants (e.g., treating physician, teacher). A critical examination of the power relationship between researcher and participant is especially relevant, in order to assess the potential for coercion. As a responsible researcher, you need to assure participants that their involvement in the study will in no way affect their access to services or the quality of their care.

Risks and Benefits

A section on the risks and benefits of the research should reflect how the participants, as well as other communities, may be affected by the research. A description of how risks and benefits will be balanced and an explanation of the strategies in place to minimize/manage risks should be included. It is important to be honest about risks and to genuinely reflect upon how to minimize them. For instance, it might be important to consider:

- Are there supports available for participants who may experience emotional distress following an interview about their experiences of living with cancer?
- Are there built-in mechanisms for dealing with research results that might be negative or unflattering to participants?
- Are there clear processes in place for ensuring that the benefits of the research will be distributed fairly and equitably between research partners?

Privacy and Confidentiality

Privacy and confidentiality are also included in the ethics protocol. This section needs to include a description of how the participants' anonymity will be maintained throughout the research, should they wish to remain anonymous. Even if some participants may wish to discuss their participation in the research with others, the researcher remains responsible for ensuring that mechanisms are in place to ensure privacy and confidentiality to all research participants. This section of the protocol must provide a detailed description of how the data will be stored, secured, and used. Important questions to consider are:

- What rules exist for working with transcripts or surveys that include identifying information?
- How are boundaries maintained between multiple roles (e.g., as researchers, health professionals, counsellors, and peers)?
- What processes are in place to be inclusive about data analysis yet maintain the privacy of research participants?
- Where will the data be kept and who will have access to it?

Compensation

Compensation is also an important aspect to consider. Any reimbursement, remuneration, or other forms of compensation that will be provided to the participants or to advisory group members should be described. Questions to guide this process might include:

- Is it important to reimburse people for their time and to honour their efforts?
- Might participants who have limited financial resources perceive the honorarium as coercive?
- Who is managing the research budget (e.g., university-based researcher, research partner in a community based agency)?
- Which partners are compensated?
- Who is being paid, who is volunteering, and how are these decisions being made?

It is essential to have clear guidelines for decision-making about compensation to ensure transparency and consistency throughout the research.

Conflict of Interest

Conflicts of interest also need to be carefully thought through and described in the ethics protocol. Providing information related to actual or potential conflicts of interest in the study will allow the ethical review board to assess whether the participants require additional information to give truly informed consent. Questions for reflection:

- What happens when the research position depends on the results of the research?
- What happens when the researcher is also a friend, peer, service provider, doctor, nurse, social worker, educator, and/or funder?
- Might the research be compromised if the researcher has multiple roles?

The procedures that will be used to obtain informed consent must be included in an ethics protocol. Typically, a copy of the information letter and consent form that will be given to the research participants is submitted. Any reasons why informed consent might not be possible or desired should also be documented. When minors are to be included as participants, a copy of the assent script to be used is also provided in the ethics submission. Questions for reflection:

- What does informed consent really mean for vulnerable populations (e.g., children, people with disabilities)?
- What meanings does consent have in different cultures?

As Tuhiwai Smith suggests,

> Asking directly for consent to interview can also be interpreted as quite rude behaviour in some cultures. Consent is not so much given for a project or specific set of questions, but for a person, for their credibility. Consent indicates trust and the assumption is that the trust will not only be reciprocated but constantly negotiated – a dynamic relationship rather than a static decision. (1999, p. 136)

Similarly, it is important to ask: What does it mean to inform? What does it mean to consent? Whose permission do I need to talk to whom?

The elements to include in an ethics protocol chart the path that will be undertaken through the participatory research process. Although participatory research in health is building momentum in Canada, it is still an approach to research that is not well understood among members of some ethical review boards. Limited expertise may lead to challenges in obtaining ethical approval for participatory research projects.

Hospital ethical review boards, which are more accustomed to appraising biomedical research and clinical trials, may not fully understand the ethical considerations in this approach. For example, because recruitment of participants from community settings is undertaken over a longer period of time than clinical studies within an already established patient population, ethical review boards may not understand why the research cannot be completed in a shorter time frame. Similarly, they may not be sufficiently well versed in qualitative methodologies to comprehend the meaning and importance of the analytic practices involved in this work. Because the health research field is so vast, it is critical to have members of diverse disciplines represented on ethical review boards, so that different studies and approaches can be evaluated fairly. I also feel strongly that patients or community members with an interest in the research should be invited to participate in ethical review boards as a matter of standard practice in hospitals and universities.

Negotiating Competing Interests – Working the Balance

My experiences conducting participatory research have revealed unexpected subtleties and complexities in maintaining research ethics and personal and professional integrity. A difficult tension in participatory research is between the desire to do *social good* with and on behalf of marginalized communities, and the fact that, as a researcher, I experience privileges, due to education, income, and living free from cancer, for example, that have placed me very differently in social hierarchies from those with whom I work (Drew, Sonn, Bishop, & Contos, 2000). It is important to see the nuances of power between differentially positioned community partners in order to find a way of doing participatory research in a socially responsible manner. With this in mind, Drew et al. propose that researchers from dominant groups

> must maintain the pain of uncertainty and ambiguity to avoid being captured by the sense of 'doing good.' The ambiguity and uncertainty serves to remind us that we are, in a sense, interlopers with the opportunity to retreat to the comfort of the dominant society when things become difficult, in the smug belief that we have helped the Indigenous community. (p. 182)

This is only one example of how privilege can operate. However, it illustrates a broader ethical dilemma in participatory research that is essential to consider, to discuss openly, and to attempt to work through.

A related concern is that research can be misrepresented, misread, or misused. What happens when research further exacerbates a social problem by turning the participants into the problem rather than illuminating the social, political, or economic causes of their life experiences? In my work with marginalized women living with breast cancer, I have been confronted with this ethical dilemma. Rather than individualizing the issues research participants are facing, I have wanted to show how structural inequalities are experienced very personally in the day to day lives of the women I have interviewed. I have needed to negotiate the competing interests at stake during every stage of the research. Sometimes research funders have ideas about how the research should be presented. These ideas may conflict with the way the research advisory committee, or the researcher, would like to present the work. Who has the power to define the ethical way forward? While I often struggle with the knowledge that there is no single path of action, I am committed to the process of collectively and individually creating options that have the potential to produce equitable results. These conflicts can be excruciatingly difficult to manage, but I am comforted in knowing that, 'to inform the decisions of where we should place our footsteps, we have only our deepest moral intuitions and the sage advice of others to act as markers in guiding our path' (Rosa, 1997).

Conclusion

Audre Lorde, a Black lesbian feminist poet and activist, taught us that 'the master's tools will never dismantle the master's house' (1979). In our work at OBCCRI we often adapt standard research tools, while incorporating more inclusive, participatory methods, towards the goal of meaningful and lasting social change. In my view, critical and reflexive approaches enable researchers to acknowledge and work from our own partial and limited perspectives based on our social positions in relation to the complex web of power and privilege in society, and from our various experiences of voice and silence throughout the research process. More concretely, this means that we make ourselves vulnerable and open to critical scrutiny, while explicitly stating our intentions and attempting to move forward in the areas where we can see opportunities for innovative ethical action and inquiry. These broader considerations are what make the ethical review process come to life, and what make ethical research possible. I hope that by making explicit some of the processes involved in doing collaborative research, and openly sharing the tensions, complexities, and meaningful moments in our work, I can work with others to build a culture of research that promotes equity.

Acknowledgments

FRANCOPHONE WOMEN WITH BREAST CANCER STUDY
Principal Investigator: Stephanie Austin
Advisory Group Members: Lucie Chauvette, Anemia Institute; Carol Burnham Cook, Willow Breast Cancer Support and Resource Services; Claire Parrot, Rouge Valley Health Systems; Simone Durantet, Centre medico-social communautaire; Manon Labrecque, Ontario Breast Cancer Community Research Initiative.

This project was funded by the Ontario Breast Cancer Community Research Initiative, which is funded by the Canadian Breast Cancer Foundation, Ontario Chapter.

REFERENCES

Austin, S. (2004). Une étude sur le vécu des femmes francophones atteintes du cancer du sein. Special issue on women's health and well-being. *Canadian Woman Studies/Cahiers de la femme, 24*(1), 43–6.
Canada. Medical Research Council of Canada, Natural Sciences and Engineering Research Council of Canada, Social Sciences and Humanities Research Council of Canada. (2003). *Tri-council policy statement: Ethical conduct for research involving humans.* Public Works and Government Services Canada. Catalogue No: MR21-18/2003E.
Carroll, W. (Ed.). (2004). *Critical strategies for social research* (pp. 262–75). Toronto, ON: Canadian Scholars' Press.
Drew, N., Sonn, C., Bishop, B., & Contos, N. (2000). 'Is doing good just enough?' Enabling practice in a disabling discipline. In T. Sloan (Ed.), *Critical psychology: Voices for change* (pp. 171–83). New York, NY: St Martin's Press.
Haraway, D.J. (1991). Situated knowledges: The science question in feminism and the privilege of partial perspective. In *Simians, cyborgs, and woman: The reinvention of nature* (pp. 183–201). New York: Routledge.
Kirby, S., Greaves, L., & Reid, C. (2006). *Experience, research, social change: Methods beyond the mainstream.* Toronto, ON: Broadview Press.

Lorde, A. (1979). The master's tools will never dismantle the master's house. Comments at 'The personal and the political' panel, Second Sex Conference.

Moosa-Mitha, M. (2005). Situating anti-oppressive theories within critical and difference-centred perspectives. In L. Brown & S. Strega (Eds.), *Research as resistance: Critical, indigenous, and anti-oppressive approaches* (pp. 237–54). Toronto, ON: Canadian Scholars' Press.

Muzychka, M., & Poulin, C. (1995). *Feminist research ethics: A process.* Ottawa: CRIAW.

Reitsma-Street, M., & Brown, L. (2004). Community action research. In W. Carroll (Ed.), *Critical strategies for social research* (pp. 303–19). Toronto, ON: Canadian Scholars' Press.

Ristock, J.L., & Pennell, J. (1996). *Community research as empowerment: Feminist links, postmodern interruptions.* Toronto, ON: Oxford University Press.

Rosa, A. (1997). *The courage to change: Salvadoran stories of personal and social transformation.* Unpublished master's thesis, Wilfrid Laurier University, Waterloo, Ontario, Canada.

Rosa, A., Russell, J., & Prilleltensky, I. (1996, August). *Social justice in community psychology.* Paper presented at the meeting of the American Psychological Association, Toronto, Canada.

St. Denis, V. (2004). Community-based participatory research: Aspects of the concept relevant for practice. In W. Carroll (Ed.), *Critical strategies for social research* (pp. 292–302). Toronto, ON: Canadian Scholars' Press.

Tuhiwai Smith, L. (1999). *Decolonizing methodologies: Research and indigenous peoples.* New York, NY: Zed Books.

3 Community Building versus Career-Building Research: The Challenges, Risks, and Responsibilities of Conducting Research with Aboriginal and Native American Communities

TERRY MITCHELL AND EMERANCE BAKER

The following chapter provides a Native and non-Native perspective on community-based participatory research with Native communities. We introduce significant challenges and discuss strategies employed to negotiate and address these challenges from an ethical and anticolonial standpoint. We emphasize the importance of ensuring that participatory research serves the interests and needs of the Native communities in which the research is being conducted. Clearer guidelines are recommended for conducting participatory research to increase the probability of researchers (Native and non-Native) successfully engaging in community-building versus career-building research.

The Aboriginal Women's Cancer Care Project (AWCCP) was designed to increase understanding of the intersection of culture, identity, and health systems in Aboriginal and Native American women's experience of and access to cancer care (see table 3, page 57). We are investigating health and cancer beliefs, decisions, and healthcare experiences of Canadian Aboriginal and Native American women with breast and gynecological cancer. This exploratory qualitative study was designed to bring women's experiences into focus to inform policy changes that address existing health disparities. In light of the many methodological challenges faced to date, in this article we discuss the emergent challenges, risks, and responsibilities within research partnerships between researchers and Aboriginal and Native American communities.

We discuss the ideals of participatory action research (PAR) and the

Table 3

ABORIGINAL IDENTITY AND WOMEN'S CANCERS

Why was the research completed?
- Aboriginal Canadians die earlier than non-Aboriginal Canadians and have a greater burden of physical disease that is inextricably linked to their socioeconomic status and history of oppression (Canadian Institute of Child Health, 1989; Canada, 1996).
- Native cancer patients continue to have the poorest five year survival rates from cancer in relation to the general population and when compared with other minority, poor, and medically underserved populations (Burhansstipanov et al., 2001; Marrett & Chaudhry, 2003).
- Though rates of breast cancer are lower in Aboriginal communities compared to the general population (Burhansstipanov et al., 2001; Marrett & Chaudhry, 2003), the age standardized cervical cancer mortality rate (per 100,000) among Ontario Status Indian women is 7.38 as compared to 3.63 among the Ontario general population of women (Marrett & Chaudhry, 2003).

What methods were used?
An Aboriginal Women's Cancer Care Project committee was formed. This committee and the project researchers investigated health and cancer beliefs, decisions, and healthcare experiences of Canadian Aboriginal and Native American women with breast and gynecological cancer. Three community-based interviewers conducted ten qualitative interviews with women with breast or gynecological cancer from four culturally and geographically diverse Aboriginal communities. Thematic analysis was utilized to identify project findings.

What were the key findings?
Key concerns identified include:

- Silence around speaking about cancer
- Health literacy
- Lag time between diagnosis and treatment
- Balance of traditional and Western treatments
- Finances
- Co-morbidities
- Lack of community cancer systems and resources
- Lack of culturally specific cancer services/supports

> **What are some implications or results of the research?**
> Existing barriers to accessible cancer care included geographical
> distance, finances, co-morbidity, beliefs and fears about cancer, the
> variable quality of health communications, compounded by silences and
> lack of support at the level of the family, community, and health system.
> Aboriginal cancer survivors and healthcare providers identified the need
> for communication and support that may break the existing silence
> around cancer. Cancer materials need to be culturally and literacy-level
> appropriate and healthcare providers need to be informed about and
> appreciate the use of traditional medicines (or, potentially, with Western
> medicines) in Aboriginal cancer care.
>
> See references at end of chapter for sources.

newly asserted research principles of community: ownership, control,
access, and possession (OCAP) of the research process and data. We
identify that PAR and OCAP provide essential principles as guidelines that are necessary but not always sufficient for successful research
collaborations. By contextualizing the research process from both the
subject position of non-Native and Native researcher, we reveal the
complexity of the research relationship and the dynamic issues of identity, trust, power, and sovereignty as negotiated in this cancer study.

Issues of History, Power, Methodology, and Ethics

Participatory Action Research

Participatory Action Research (PAR) is defined as 'systematic inquiry,
with the collaboration of those affected by the issues being studied,
for purposes of education and taking action or effecting social change'
(Green, George, Daniel, & Frankish, 1995). PAR methods are viewed as
appropriate and increasingly essential in conducting research with vulnerable, hard to reach, or medically underserved populations. PAR is
viewed as appropriate because the research values are empowering and
restorative and because of the explicit commitment that the outcomes
should benefit the participants and/or their communities (Chrisman,
Strickland, Powell, Squeochs, & Yallup, 1999). PAR is conceptualized as
a research approach that will promote the mutual production of knowl-

edge: knowledge that is liberating rather than oppressive, knowledge that reveals and challenges systemic problems rather than reinforcing relations of dominance.

Implicit in PAR is a balance of risks and benefits that should favour the needs and well-being of the participants over the researchers. PAR is an idealistic, values-based, liberatory approach to research with an explicit empowerment mandate (Park, 1993). The research is usually conducted with and for the use of marginalized or oppressed groups. The goal is to improve participant lives through structural change. The research issue is to be identified by and/or with the community, and community members are ideally involved in contributing to the entire research process, which strengthens participants' awareness of their own strengths while building skills and knowledge in a collaborative process that supports change (Hall, 1981).

Despite the explicit values of PAR to partner with and advocate for a group of marginalized or disenfranchised people, the practice of PAR is not explicit. Although there are guidelines, such as ongoing involvement of participants throughout all stages of the research, there are no clear guidelines as to how the ongoing research relationship is to be developed or how one negotiates power issues within the field. There are few if any guidelines on how power relations can either be reinforced or reshaped through PAR. What is known is largely unwritten and may ultimately be context specific. This has led to perceived and actual abuses by conventional researchers working under the PAR mantle to gain entry to communities and access to insider knowledge while still maintaining researcher control of the processes and the products of the research (Hagey, 1997).

The Research Chill

Canadian Aboriginal and Native American communities are increasingly wary of external researchers, expressing concern that they are being 'researched to death' (Schnarch, 2004). Epidemiological studies, for example, have depicted Aboriginal and Native American peoples as sick, powerless, and lacking in capacity, information that is used to reinforce unequal power relations, paternalism, and dominance, and to undermine their aspirations for sovereignty (O'Neil, Reading, & Leader, 1998). Approaching Aboriginal and Native American communities with PAR studies as a means of engaging them in research partnerships is insufficient to counterbalance the many harms created by outsider research; however, it is an important start in this process. Partnerships are more astutely understood by many Aboriginal and Native American communities as a 'euphemism' for a relationship of individuals with unequal amounts of power and an uncertain balance of risks and benefits that most often favours external researchers (O'Neil et al.).

It is clear that Western methodologies and institutional ethics processes are not enough to ensure the integrity, validity, and ethical nature of research in Aboriginal and Native American communities. Conventional academic research interests and methodologies and Aboriginal and Native American research interests and traditional forms of knowing do not make a natural fit. The clash between Aboriginal philosophies and positivist science has been described as 'jagged worldviews colliding' (Castellano, 2004).

However, Aboriginal and Native American communities have an increasing need for complementarity of methodologies, for an intercultural lens that ensures both the trustworthiness of research at the community level and external credibility to inform policy and access funding (Castellano). With increasing attention to political processes of self-governance and sovereignty, Aboriginal and Native American communities are taking control of ethical review processes and decisions about which research does or does not happen in their communities. This means that researchers approaching Native American and Aboriginal communities for approval of research projects can be met with considerable scepticism, often waiting months for community approval with a very low success rate (O'Neil et al., 1998). This positive move towards increased sovereignty has resulted in a potential slowdown or 'chill' on research until clearer partnership guidelines and practices are established (Castellano).

Principles of Research in Canadian Aboriginal Communities: OCAP

Increased sovereignty is expressed in part by increased control of community research. OCAP is a recently coined acronym (Schnarch, 2004), which is a synthesis of proposed responses to grievances that have been advanced by Canadian Aboriginal peoples for many years. OCAP is a set of principles developed to ensure ethical and beneficial research that conforms to the cultures and needs of Aboriginal communities and serves to value and preserve Indigenous knowledge bases. It is part of a restorative process in which Aboriginal research plays a major role in restoring power and control to Aboriginal communities and individuals (Schnarch). The AWCCP is guided by the principles of OCAP to ensure that our research practices are in keeping with the laws, values, and ethics of the Aboriginal and Native American communities in which we are working, and to redress the power imbalances common in much of the prior research done 'for' or 'about' communities. However, OCAP is a 'set of principles in evolution,' not an Aboriginal methodology (Schnarch). This is a salient point when considering the current challenges of implementing the principles of OCAP within mainstream academic research.

In the rest of the chapter, we describe our research project and how we experienced, as Native and non-Native researchers, both the embrace and chill of communities in relation to collaborative research. We describe our processes and our research challenges and the strategies we employed to negotiate these challenges. These challenges are in no way unique or comprehensive. We have, within the scope of this chapter, attempted to address those issues that were most salient: identity and subject location, development of community research partnerships, parameters of consent, control of data and participant privacy, and the vagaries of time within community-based research.

Aboriginal Women's Cancer Care Project

We chose a PAR model of community-based research in which members of the research population are involved at all stages of the research process in various paid and unpaid roles. The AWCCP is an ongoing collaborative community research project in which the co-principal investigators of this study are a non-Aboriginal Canadian assistant professor (TM) and a Native American retired academic and director of a national cancer research centre (EB). The study is coordinated by an Aboriginal project coordinator and guided by an Aboriginal and Native American advisory group (six individuals from five different communities: Inuit, Mohawk, and Ojibway).

The AWCCP attempted to conduct research with five culturally and geographically different communities including two reservation communities, an off-reserve urban population, and with Inuit women who were travelling from their northern communities for health services in an urban centre. We are attempting to conduct in-depth, individual, open-ended qualitative interviews with six cancer survivors, two family members, and two healthcare practitioners in each community. The participants are self-identified Aboriginal and Native American women, their family members, and healthcare providers who belong to northern, urban, rural, or reservation communities.

Key Challenges and Strategies

What is largely absent from the literature are the realities, vulnerabilities, and emotional risks that each partner faces when negotiating research partnerships. Although successful research collaborations, by community standards, have been forged between external researchers and Native American communities, the trust between community and research partners is at best tenuous due in large part to the history of exploitation of Aboriginal and Native American communities by governments and research institutions. These issues of trust, however, are not always one-sided or fixed, as trust and participation are 'conditional' and 'fluid' conditions of any research process (Elias, O'Neil, & Sanderson, 2004). As we reflect on the emerging challenges, risks, responsibilities, and conundrums in developing and maintaining long-term research partnerships with Aboriginal and Native American communities, we consider our own subject locations and how they influence and are impacted by the project processes and outcomes.

Identity and Subject Location: Two Voices

No one has a pure world view that is 100 per cent Indigenous or Eurocentric; rather, everyone has an integrated mind, a fluxing and ambidextrous consciousness, a pre-colonized consciousness that flows into a colonized consciousness and back again (Little Bear, 2000). As a non-Native woman (author TM), it has been my honour and my challenge to conduct collaborative research with Aboriginal communities at different times over the past thirteen years. Issues of history, identity, voice, oppression, resistance, and transformation are constant. I have been welcomed, and I have been scorned, trusted and mistrusted, often in cyclical patterns that resonate most strongly with potent histories rather than, I believe, with personal acts or contemporary relations.

Although Castellano theorized about the chill in Aboriginal research and the current need to try to face challenges to continue to form collaborative research relationships with non-Natives, the very material risk of not 'making it' as an Aboriginal researcher working in Aboriginal and Native American communities is not mentioned. This is not uncommon; challenges have been documented for entry and acceptance of non-Native researchers (Little Bear). However, the identity, trust, and entry issues experienced by Aboriginal and Native American researchers have rarely been acknowledged. My own location (author EB) as an Aboriginal researcher often entails a hypervigilance in both the academic and Aboriginal research communities. It is a constant balancing act in which there is little room for error and even less space for both world views to play out successfully.

In the academic culture, there is still an expectation (obvious in most of the published literature on 'capacity building') that most or all of the capacity building in Aboriginal research is intended for or directed to the community. As an Aboriginal researcher working in both cultures, it is clear that academic and funding institutions are generally lacking in policy and practices required for conducting Aboriginal research. Conducting ethical Aboriginal research requires attention to bi-directional learning and capacity building.

STRATEGIES

When asked why, as Native and non-Native researchers, we would be willing to work in such a demanding research environment, we came to realize there is no other way for us to do ethical community research. Our intercultural partnership provides us with perspective and support when faced with challenges linked to race and identity. Although the principles and practices of OCAP and PAR offer significant challenges to researchers, we believe that they also produce significantly more credible and beneficial research by, for, and about communities and individuals. We are working interculturally to form dialogue and support around the challenges of community-building research. Making the tensions conscious and sharing them first with each other and then with the research community is a strategy to address the inherent challenges of conducting research in Native American and Canadian Aboriginal communities.

Developing Community Research Partnerships

A major challenge was trying to partner with geographically and culturally different communities. Whereas many granting agencies, universities, and Aboriginal and Native American communities are striving to establish best practices of research in Native American and Aboriginal communities (Castellano), guidelines and published accounts of research experience in conducting research in this context are still limited.

For the AWCCP, each community partner had specific ethics protocols for conducting research in their community. The processes for ethics approval varied from community to community as did the manner in which researchers should approach the community itself before an ethics protocol was submitted. In one instance, the AWCCP research coordinator erroneously approached the community health advisory board first, as she had been informed of this process in approaching a community previously. Because she had breached the approach protocol with this community – by not going to band council first – she was suspected of trying to circumvent their ethics process. In another community, the project coordinator approached the band council first to discover that the health council was sceptical of her ability to work honestly with them, as they were to be approached first in that particular community. Although the band council did approve the AWCCP in that community, it took a concerted effort to reestablish the trust with the health council – which ultimately oversaw research in their community.

STRATEGIES

Although we are working through and continually managing these challenges in respectful ways, there is still the process of rebuilding a very fragile community trust involved with perceived and actual breaches of community protocols. Ultimately, we developed and submitted six ethics research protocols; one for each community/institutional partner. We submitted ethics protocols for Wilfrid Laurier University; Sunnybrook and Women's College Health Sciences Centre; Akwesasne New York; and Curve Lake First Nation, Ontario, as well as an application to the Nunavut Research Institute and to the first reserve community. Ethics review processes varied between two weeks, two months, and two years across the different communities. All, except the original reserve community, have now approved the project, and the AWCCP is proceeding through each of its iterative stages in these communities.

Individual or Community: Who Has the Authority to Give Consent?

The AWCCP has undergone numerous changes as a direct response to the challenges encountered as both a collaborative and participatory project. In our research process, we have experienced challenges in which the principles of OCAP and the laws and values of the community partners are in direct conflict with the individual wishes of community members. It was made clear to us through a number of individuals who were concerned about their own autonomy and rights being suppressed for the 'good' of the community that consent is a complicated issue that is negotiated with individuals, groups, or communities. Conventionally, consent is established with individuals; however, in this study, we acknowledged the sovereignty of communities by not interviewing individuals from a community that did not provide ethics approval. A research challenge arose when several individuals (cancer survivors, a family member, and a healer) questioned our decision to abide by the decision of their community's ethics council.

STRATEGIES

Our response to this challenge emerged from consultation with our advisory group, who guided us to respect the sovereignty and governance of the local community by not, for example, interviewing individual cancer survivors off reserve. We decided not to include the members of the cancer survivors group and other cancer survivors who asked to be interviewed as research participants in the AWCCP. However, this decision to build research partnerships with communities versus individuals, and, by so doing, to respect the sovereignty of communities, did not diminish the individual survivors' feelings of being excluded and silenced. The development of an emerging community research methodology needs to attend to the power and control issues within the communities themselves as well as between the researchers and Aboriginal and Native American communities. Although the conundrum of individual versus community consent needs to be acknowledged and respected by researchers, we do not believe that the academic/research community should attempt to address or circumvent these issues, which are in the domain of the communities themselves.

Privacy and Confidentiality of Data

Another challenge is ensuring the protection of participants' rights to privacy and confidentiality. Access to and ownership of research data, as outlined in OCAP, is increasingly a primary concern for band councils in Canada and tribal groups in the United States. Community ethics protocols request that communities have access to and possession of all raw project data. The management of the confidentiality of sensitive cancer experience data is a serious responsibility of researchers. Data storage and security must be agreed on in the written consent obtained from each participant.

STRATEGIES

Therefore, when a community explicitly requested to store all raw data in their community archive, we negotiated a middle ground with the community. First, we confirmed that we understood and supported the community's right to access and ownership of all findings but raised our concern that storage of confidential tapes and transcripts would have to be the choice of the individual research participants. We were aware that, despite the principles of OCAP, some individuals might not wish their personal transcripts to be stored in their own community. We developed a process regarding access that we believed was respectful of the community's request, a response that was transparent and clear, one that indicated that access to the data would be stage dependent and that ownership of the data would remain with the participants.

The community accepted our proposed solution that at differing stages the form of the data would change and that access to data would change accordingly. We proposed that when the data is raw in the form of audio tapes and transcribed interviews, access is reduced to the interviewers, the participants, the transcriber, and the primary investigators. When the data is at the second stage, any identifying markers are removed through a process of *member checking* in which interviewers review an individual's transcripts with the individual research participants for correctness of the data and privacy of the participant. The data can then be accessed by the larger research group. In the third stage, in which the data is analysed and thematically organized into findings, access expands to include the advisory group, the Aboriginal community (including chief and council), and the larger research community. Ultimately, it is the consent of the participants that determines whether their personal raw data will be stored with the researcher or their community.

Research Takes Time

In 2001, I (author TM) made links with an Aboriginal cancer support group from the first reservation community. The support group met with me off reserve and expressed the desire to share their stories of survival and hope with other Aboriginal communities. They discussed the possibility of conducting interviews that would lead to the development of a radio drama. Funding was sought and received for an exploratory study, and I obtained an ethics review at my university. I made regular trips to the community to join the survivors group at their meetings. Ethics materials were reviewed and discussed and were left with the group members to review over the next month before signing. I returned to the community the following month to obtain consent and to discuss funding and hiring issues for the project with the survivors group. After one and a half years of working with this group (but never collecting any data), I was abruptly informed at another meeting in the community that I had breached all research protocols and must now seek approval from the community's ethics review council before proceeding. I learned this for the first time despite having explicitly asked at the first and subsequent survivor group meetings if permission of chief and council was required.

STRATEGIES

I then chose to begin at the beginning to redress any perceived or actual breaches of protocol. I established an Aboriginal advisory group with representatives from six different communities, including two from the survivor support group's community, which included a member from the survivor support group.

Time remains a challenge. We have had limited success in recruiting research participants (n=10), and we have not conducted interviews with the original survivors group or interviewed individual survivors who live in the community where we did not gain band council approval. However, after two and a half years, the AWCCP has had significant achievements in building the foundation for ethical and successful research partnerships. We have developed a strong Aboriginal advisory group with representatives from five communities, have obtained six ethics approvals, and have developed partnerships with two reservation communities. By honouring our community research partnership and the sovereignty of the community that did not grant ethics approval, we face the difficult decision of choosing to exclude the very cancer survivors who initiated this project. However, we have clarified that in conducting PAR research, informed by specific principles, our research partnerships are formed with Canadian Aboriginal and Native American communities rather than with individuals or groups. We are confident that those research partnerships are consistent with the ethical demands of OCAP: community ownership, control, access, and possession of research processes and outputs.

Lessons Learned: Community-building versus Career-building Research

We have learned that history shapes all current research relationships in one way or another. Research within Aboriginal and Native American communities is constrained and defined by the historical relations of dominance, ongoing issues of achieving sovereignty and reclaiming ownership of Indigenous knowledge, and prior experiences of negative research practices. Time is, therefore, essential in developing trust and building relationships and partnerships that are for the long-term benefit of communities collaborating in research. The primary condition of Aboriginal research is developing and maintaining right relationships (Castellano, 2004).

Right relationships refers to working in a holistic manner in developing balanced relationships that involve respect and which are developed over time. Working in Native communities requires time to build and sustain relationships – those that are not simply business or research partnerships. Research relationships are embedded in relationships which emerge out of care and respect for one another, through visiting, sharing about one's family, often over a cup of tea, a meal, or a community feast. Developing community relationships and research practices that are beneficial to Aboriginal communities requires indeterminate amounts of time. The uncertain time frame and success rate of community entry, ethics review processes, recruitment, and publication presents considerable tension for university-based researchers. Although academic researchers can provide valuable research services to communities (usually without direct payment), researchers are under considerable pressure to write and publish research findings to maintain their jobs. Capacity building and structural changes must occur at the institutional and funding levels so that funding agencies, ethics review boards, and university promotion and tenure committees are informed of and responsive to the necessity of the time needed for trust building, community entry, and the building of sustainable research relationships within an OCAP era.

We have learned that the liberatory and empowerment ideals of PAR are not enough and that the principles of OCAP, when conducting research in partnership with Aboriginal communities, are essential but not yet adequately articulated in practice. Clearer guidelines, combined with practice examples and lessons learned from the field, will be important in shaping future research collaborations between researchers and Aboriginal and Native American communities. The difficulty in engaging OCAP principles is shaped by the dissonance between OCAP and the demands/constraints of mainstream research institutions. Although negotiating the principles of OCAP into the day to day practices of Aboriginal and Native American research is time consuming and fraught with perils for Native and non-Native researchers alike, authentic PAR informed by OCAP shifts existing power relations and recalibrates the balance of risks and benefits for researchers and communities.

Acknowledgments

The authors acknowledge the cancer survivors, their loved ones, and community healthcare providers who have shared their voices and their stories to improve cancer care for themselves and for their communities. The authors thank the community members who took the time to review their ethics proposal regardless of the outcome. The authors express their deepest appreciation for the gifts of guidance and support from the members of their advisory group – Linda Burhansstipanov, Doris Cook, Katherine Gofton, Barb Harris, Paul Skanks, Valorie Whetung, and RoseAnne Wyman – without whom they would not have the understanding of community partnerships necessary to proceed.

This project was one of three projects of the Intersecting Vulnerabilities research program, which was funded by the Canadian Institutes of Health Research. The Canadian Breast Cancer Foundation, Ontario Chapter funds the Ontario Breast Cancer Community Research Initiative, home of the Intersecting Vulnerabilities research program.

A version of this chapter was published in *Journal of Cancer Education* Special Supplement, Vol. 20, Spring 2005, pp. 41–6. It is reprinted with permission from Lawrence Erlbaum Associates.

REFERENCES

Burhansstipanov, L., Gilbert, A., LaMarca, K., & Krebs, L.U. (2001). An innovative path to improving cancer care in Indian country. *Public Health Reports, 116*, 424–33.

Canada. (1996). Royal Commission on Aboriginal Peoples. *Report of the Royal Commission on Aboriginal Peoples*. Ottawa: Canada Communications Group Publishing.

Canadian Institute of Child Health. (1989). *The health of Canada's children: A CICH profile*. Ottawa: Canadian Institute of Child Health.

Castellano, M.B. (2004). Ethics of Aboriginal research. *Journal of Aboriginal Health, 1*, 98–114.

Chrisman, N.J., Strickland, C.J., Powell, K., Squeochs, M.D., & Yallup, M. (1999). Community partnership research with the Yakama Indian Nation. *Human Organization, 58*, 134–41.

Elias, B., O'Neil, J.D., & Sanderson, D. (2004). The politics of trust and participation: A case study of developing First Nations and university capacity to build health information systems in a First Nations context. *Journal of Aboriginal Health, 1*, 68–78.

Green, L., George, M., Daniel, M., & Frankish, C. (1995). *Study of participatory research in health promotion: Review and recommendations for the development of participatory research in health promotion in Canada by the Institute of Health Promotion Research, University of British Columbia & B.C. Consortium for Health Promotion*. Ottawa, Ontario: Royal Society of Canada.

Hagey, R.S. (1997). The use and abuse of participatory action research. *Chronic Diseases in Canada, 18*, 1–6.

Hall, B. (1981). Participatory research, popular knowledge and power: A personal reflection. *Convergence: An International Journal of Adult Education, 14*, 6–19.

Little Bear, L. (2000). Jagged worldviews colliding. In M. Battiste (Ed.), *Reclaiming indigenous voice and vision* (p. 85). Vancouver: UBC Press.

Marrett, L.D., & Chaudhry, M. (2003). Cancer incidence and mortality in Ontario First Nations, 1968–1991 (Canada). *Cancer Causes and Control, 14*(3), 259–68.

O'Neil, J.D., Reading, J.R., & Leader, A. (1998). Changing the relations of surveillance: The development of a discourse of resistance in Aboriginal epidemiology. *Human Organization, 57*, 230–7.

Park, P. (1993). What is participatory research? A theoretical and methodological perspective. In P. Park, M. Brydon-Miller, B. Hall, and T. Jackson (Eds.), *Voices of change: Participatory research in the United States and Canada* (pp. 1–20). Toronto, Ontario: Greenwood Publishing Group.

Schnarch, B. (2004). Ownership, control, access and possession (OCAP) or self-determination applied to research: A critical analysis of contemporary first nations research and some options for first nation communities. *Journal of Aboriginal Health, 1,* 80–95.

PART TWO

Approaches in Data Analysis

4 Listening for Echoes: How Social Location Matters in Women's Experiences of Cancer Care

JUDY GOULD, CHRIS SINDING, TERRY MITCHELL, AND
MARGARET I. FITCH

The Intersecting Vulnerabilities research program began with the separate investigations by three research teams of the cancer care experiences of Aboriginal women (led by author TM), older women (led by author CS), and lower-income women (led by JG). We focused on the lived experience of breast or gynecological cancer among women who occupy these three social locations as critical cases – critical sites for knowledge development about women's gendered experiences of health, illness, and care. A second phase of the project explored women's similar experiences across the communities.

The main focus of the research was to understand how interactions with the health system can both contribute to and alleviate social and health disparities among women from vulnerable populations.

Patterns of Health System Access among Lower-income, Older, and Aboriginal Women

Though 'health services' is listed as a social determinant of health it is not granted high status (Canada, Federal, Provincial and Territorial Advisory Committee on Population Health, 1996). The interaction of health services with other social determinants of health such as income, age, and Aboriginal status was the focus of this investigation.

Lower-income Women with Breast Cancer (see table 4, page 76)

The five-year breast cancer survival rate for women with household incomes of less than $20,000U.S. per year is 64 per cent compared to 76

Table 4

Lower-Income Women with Breast Cancer

Why was the research completed?
The five-year survival rate for women with household incomes of less
than $20,000/year is 64 per cent, compared to 76 per cent for women
with household incomes of over $50,000/year (Mackillop et al., 1997).
- Explanations for higher risk of death include that lower-income women
  have higher rates of co-morbidity (Kasper, 2002) and are more likely
  to present with advanced cancers than higher-income women (Farley
  & Flannery, 1989).
- Presenting later with cancer, however, does not account fully for higher mortality rates. Mackillop et al. (1997) posit that 'although Canada's
  health care system was designed to provide equitable access to
  equivalent standards of care it does not prevent a difference in cancer
  survival between rich and poor communities' (p. 1680).
Though the literature on the inverse relationship between breast cancer
mortality rates and socioeconomic status in Canada has been well
established (Lannin et al., 1998; Macleod et al., 2000), the experience of
breast cancer from the perspective of lower-income women is less well
understood.

What methods were used?
Fourteen women who lived below the Low Income Cut Off (Canada's
unofficial poverty line), and who had breast cancer, were interviewed
about the financial experience associated with having breast cancer
treatment. Patterns of meaning in the transcripts were identified using
content analysis.

What were the key findings?
Women experienced:
- Difficulties securing money from public and private insurance
  systems
- Lack of connection/knowledge of cancer care resources
- Financial hardship brought on by transportation, parking, and
  medication fees
- Increased ability to negotiate the cancer system if they had relation-
  ships with health professionals

What are some implications or results of the research?
- This pilot work was the foundation for research with cancer health

professionals on barriers and facilitators associated with the financial experience of lower-income women with breast cancer.
• The cancer centre involved with this research is now investigating ways to connect all new patients with drug reimbursement strategies/ support around financial issues.

See references at end of chapter for sources.

per cent for women with household incomes of over $50,000 per year (Mackillop, Zhang-Salomons, Groome, Paszat, & Holowaty, 1997). In one study with a sample of over 10,000 patients, researchers concluded that, while lower-income women took longer to seek medical attention, stage differences at diagnosis could not fully explain differences in mortality (Karjalainen & Pukkala, 1990). Some argue that differing mortality rates reflect systemic practices in healthcare (Wang & Arnold, 2002). Lower-income patients more often encounter difficult interactions with healthcare providers than their higher-income counterparts (Lannin et al., 1998).

Canadian evidence further suggests that restructuring has left the health system unresponsive to changing distributions of health needs in the population (Eyles, Birch, & Newbold, 1995). The restructuring of cancer treatment services to include increased outpatient services also increases the financial burden for individuals and families (Moore, 1999). Supportive care services are similarly patterned by broad social determinants of health. One survey conducted in Canada revealed that lower-income women with breast cancer were less likely to seek supportive care services (Gray et al., 2000). Supportive care resources tend to be especially ill-suited for people with English as a second language, those with low literacy, and those living within the lower socioeconomic brackets of society (Cancer Care Ontario, 2002; Davis, Williams, Marin, Parker, & Glass, 2002; Kagawa-Singer & Kassim-Lakha, 2003).

Older Women and Cancer (see table 5, page 78)

Along virtually every axis of the social determinants of health, older women are vulnerable: women over the age of sixty-five are almost

Table 5

OLDER WOMEN WITH BREAST CANCER

Why was the research completed?
The effect of age on patterns of cancer care is a subject of debate.
Controversy abounds, for instance, regarding appropriate medical
investigation and treatment for older people. Some researchers suggest
that older patients' generally more conservative treatment is inadequate;
others report that less aggressive treatment appropriately reflects the
diminished usefulness of systemic therapy in older people.
   Debates about how older age affects cancer care are almost always
undertaken from the perspective of health professionals and framed in
medical terms. This research sought to foreground older women's own
accounts of receiving care and treatment for cancer.

What methods were used?
Semi-structured interviews were conducted with each participant;
second interviews followed several weeks later. The interview guide
was developed by the project team with input from four additional senior
cancer survivors. The three interviewers (all in their late sixties or early
seventies; two are cancer survivors) were drawn from the project team.
In keeping with our participatory approach, each interview transcript was
reviewed and discussed by all project team members.

What were the key findings?
Study participants assessed their care extremely positively, rarely
perceiving barriers related to age or generation. Living many years
appears to affect the experience and evaluation of cancer care: age
and generation often lent participants a useful 'perspective' on cancer.
In terms of cancer care, the research showed how age-related life and
health circumstances can intersect with professional practice and wider
social contexts to affect treatment decision-making (including decisions
against treatment) as well as the day to day 'getting around' that cancer
care requires.

What are some implications or results of the research?
In discussing their cancer experience, many women compared it with
difficult things that had happened in their lives, and current pressing
health and social problems. They also valued 'getting on with things,' and
didn't want to be seen as complainers. Because of these things – other

---

> social and health problems, and the commitment not to dwell on things
> – the worries, the complaints, and the struggles that cancer brings to
> women in their seventies and eighties may disappear from view. This
> is something we need to watch for in practice and research. In cancer
> care, individual-level care and systems advocacy is required to ensure
> that older women's worries about sustaining independence (including
> worries generated by inadequacies in home-based care) do not act as
> determinants of treatment choices.

twice as likely as men to be poor (Ontario Community Support Association, 2001), they are more vulnerable to inadequate nutrition and to difficulty in accessing uninsured healthcare (Canada, Health Canada, 1999), and they often live with diminished social networks and chronic health problems that limit mobility and activities. A cancer diagnosis in an older woman's life is a health crisis that often intersects, in ways we know very little about, with precarious social and material circumstances.

More than half of new breast cancer cases in Canada occur in women sixty or over, and nearly a third in women seventy and over (Canadian Cancer Society / National Cancer Institute of Canada, 2007). The effect of age on patterns of cancer care and treatment is a subject of considerable debate. Controversy abounds, for instance, regarding appropriate medical investigation and treatment for older people (Balducci, 2001; Lickley, 1997; Turner, Haward, Mulley, & Selby, 1999; Yarborough, 2004). We know that the care of older women is less likely to be consistent with clinical guidelines than is the care of younger women (Yancik et al., 2001). Studies suggest that older women are less likely than younger women to receive extensive pre-treatment assessments (Silliman, Troyan, Guadagnoli, Kaplan, & Greenfield, 1997) and are referred to an oncologist after surgery less frequently than are younger patients (Siminoff, Zhang, Saunders Sturm, & Colabianchi, 2000). Physicians tend to spend less time with older than younger patients and are less likely to involve them in decisions (Lickley), and may be especially likely to withhold information in order to 'protect' older patients (Crooks, 2001). Older women are also less likely to be referred for clinical trials (Siminoff et al., 2000).

Some investigators suggest that older patients' generally less aggressive treatment appropriately reflects the diminished efficacy of adjuvant systemic therapy in older people (Guadagnoli et al., 1997) or the presence of significant additional health problems. However, co-morbidity does not appear to account fully for age-related variation in treatment, and the idea that older women experience more significant adverse effects from adjuvant chemotherapy has also been challenged (Watters, Yau, O'Rourke, Tomiak, & Gertler, 2003). Thus some researchers characterize older patients' more conservative investigation and treatment as 'less than ideal' (Wanebo et al., 1997); others call it 'inferior' to that of younger women (Muss, 2002), and some identify ageism as a factor in their treatment as it contrasts with that of younger women (Kearney & Miller, 2000), and in some cases explicitly link patterns of treatment for older women with breast cancer to higher rates of recurrence and mortality (Silliman, 2003).

Aboriginal Women and Cancer (see table 3, page 57)

It is well documented that Aboriginal Canadians die earlier than non-Aboriginal Canadians and have a greater burden of physical and mental disease that is inextricably linked to their socioeconomic status and history of oppression (MacMillan, MacMillan, Offord, & Dingle, 1996; Royal Commission on Aboriginal Peoples, 1996). Aboriginal populations have morbidity and mortality rates that are much higher than the general Canadian population, reinforced and compounded by poor socioeconomic conditions, particularly for those living on reserve (Macmillan et al.). The four most common cancers in Status Indian women are breast, cervix, colorectal, and lung – together these account for over half of the cancers found in Status Indian women (Marrett & Chaudhry, 2003). Aboriginal/Native women in Canada and the United States have been shown to be at higher risk for developing and dying from cancer of the cervix than the general population (Burhansstipanov, 2001). While Status Indians have at least a 40 per cent lower incidence of cancer generally than non-Aboriginal women, cervical cancer occurs a startling 73 per cent more often in Status Indian women compared to all Ontario women (Marrett & Chaudhry). Despite the existence of effective secondary preventive measures, studies have shown that the Aboriginal population is less likely than lower risk groups to participate in Papanicolau (Pap) test screening programs (Lantz et al., 2003). A large population-based study in Canada found that Pap smear rates were 30 per cent lower among Native women (Hislop, Deschamps, Band, Smith, & Clarke, 1992).

Health Disparity Research

Health disparity investigations are normally carried out within a psychosocial/biomedical research paradigm (Weber & Parra-Medina, 2003). In this approach:

- individuals are treated as units of analysis and not perceived as situated amidst social forces;
- social inequities refer to differences in the distribution of resources versus the power relationships between the haves and have-nots;
- research findings are viewed through the lens of the dominant group instead of through the lens of multiply oppressed groups;
- inequalities are seen as discrete and measurable in relationship to one another versus as intertwined and socially constructed; and,
- researchers conduct value-free science versus investing in projects to make social change (Weber & Parra-Medina, 2003).

In our work, we intended to challenge this paradigm.

The Focus of the Current Work

The current work addresses shortcomings and gaps in the current literature in the following ways. Our approach is firmly rooted in social constructionist traditions: we consider gender along with socioeconomic status, aboriginal identity, and age as *social* locations – positions in social systems of dominance and subordination, privilege and marginalization. While a considerable body of research examines associations between specific social locations and health outcomes, very little research has explored health or quality of life in relation to multiple social locations. To address multiple social locations and multiple aspects of marginalization our work focuses explicitly on the development of tools and substantive knowledge about the processes that link poverty, Aboriginal identity, and older age to quality of life, and possibly to survival in the current healthcare context. In approaching the work qualitatively, we deliberately foreground the perspectives of oppressed groups, and heed Macintyre's (1986) call for researchers to 'get behind the labels ... and explore their meaning for the everyday lives and life chances of those on whom the labels are imposed' (p. 400). Finally, our participatory approach is explicitly value-laden: our intent is to effect social change including raising awareness within the cancer care sys tem about systemic inequities which prevent the just distribution of resources.

Methodology/Analysis

The Community-specific Process

In working with 'vulnerable' social groups we decided it was appropriate to use a qualitative, inductive, and participatory action research methodology to build working relationships with identified communities and to ensure reciprocity and action for the participating communities. A qualitative, inductive approach is appropriate when little is known about a phenomenon and is particularly useful to public health research where social contexts of people's lives is of critical significance (Baum, 1995; McDonald & Daly, 1992; Morse, 1995). We employed a social-constructivist methodology (Patton, 2001) to investigate the experiences and perspectives of the members of each study population.

Participatory action research purposefully involves stakeholders in much of the research design, implementation, analysis, and dissemination. Participatory action research methods are particularly appropriate when conducting research with marginalized communities (Mitchell & Baker, 2005). PAR attempts to empower stakeholders and to be of benefit to those who participate (Minkler & Wallerstein, 2003).

Our study was designed and conducted as an interdisciplinary research project that emphasized collaboration with multiple partners. We were committed to actively including members of the study populations in the research processes through the development of population-specific advisory groups. Six iterative cycles were designed into the study: community engagement, data collection, community-specific preliminary analysis, interpretation and data collection, cross-community analysis and community feedback, and proposals for action. Data collection for the community-specific preliminary analysis included in-depth qualitative interviews conducted with each of the population groups: lower-income women (n=14), Aboriginal women (n=12), and two cycles of interviews with women aged seventy and over (n=15).

Cross-community Analysis

A central aim of this research program was to identify and articulate tools for analysing experiences across a range of marginalized social locations. The multi-discipline team (from nursing, social work, community and clinical psychology, public health sciences, health studies, Native studies, community medicine) intended to explore how social factors compromising quality of life and survival for one community mirrored the factors that affect other marginalized groups. Yet we were alert to the problems of overstating commonalities, and obscuring the particular histories and contexts of each group of women. We came to understand our task as listening for what we are calling 'echoes' or parallel experiences or processes across social locations that could be more closely examined for their specific content and social and health implications.

As community-specific analyses (detailed elsewhere in Gould, 2004; Sinding, Wiernikowski, & Aronson, 2005; Mitchell & St. Germaine-Small, 2005) were nearing completion, the cross-community analysis – from which this chapter was drawn – began in earnest. Drawing on our range of disciplinary and practice perspectives, the research team dedicated time at regular meetings to listen across the findings emerging from each of the three projects. At one meeting, for example, JG noted that the lower-income women she interviewed often spoke about how effectively they managed their finances. CS and TM echoed that this finding appeared in their data. At the same meeting CS discussed the ways participants in the older women study spoke of cancer as a relatively insignificant feature of their biographies.

Among the possible interpretations is that participants asserted valued identities (such as 'I'm a good money manager even though I am supported by the welfare state' or 'I won't complain about my cancer and bother busy health professionals') against popular discourses that construct marginalized women in negative ways. Yet these important efforts to preserve valued identities sometimes seemed to compromise entitlement to medical attention or financial assistance – a finding we wanted to explore further. Our cross-community analysis was to move forward substantially at a two-day workshop involving all investigators, two advisory group members from the Older Women project, and two graduate students.

Preparing for the Cross-community Analysis Workshop

To prepare for this workshop JG, TM, and CS met to determine how we could begin to approach the cross-community analysis with such varied data. Faced with the task of understanding how different experiences could result in or echo similar consequences for women across social locations, we resolved that we could only understand the range and depth of the data by returning once again to the women's stories. Since the focus of the data was lived experience, we wondered about the following: If the experiences differed within and between populations, would the quality of care nevertheless still be comparable? What was the flavour and texture of women's interaction with health professionals? How might we re-view the research participants' recalled experiences through the lenses of equity and marginality? To answer these questions, and with our respective data sets in mind, we settled on two themes: 'silence and voice,' 'vulnerability and resistance.' We believed these themes were reflected in our data sets and would illuminate the texture and quality of women's interactions with the health system.

By silence and voice we refer to those instances in which women deliberately muted or alternatively named their needs in relation to health professionals. Examples of silence could include those instances in which women recalled wanting to indicate a need but did not for fear of inaction or, worse, reprisal. Examples of voice included recalled or intended moments of asserting a need/relaying a decision to a health professional. Vulnerability and resistance were themes that we applied to the data to address ways in which women were affected by, and responded to, their treatments and to action(s) initiated by the health system. Health-system initiated actions typically occurred during diagnosis or follow-up appointments, surgery, and chemotherapy and radiation treatments.

In this process we did not dichotomize silence and voice or resistance and vulnerability, as often one was embedded in the other or both apparent in the same section of a transcript. For example, one woman from the low-income study recalled the following circumstance in response to receiving chemotherapy treatment:

> I had a few more months to go for the chemo, but I couldn't take the rest of it, it was making me feel sick [vulnerability] and I just decide[d] after I got sick ... at work, I decided, that's it, no more chemo [vulnerability and resistance].

We felt that her need to ensure that she did not miss work (her vulnerability) rendered the 'choice' to refuse (resist) treatment questionable. In other words, it appeared to us that her financial situation made for a situation with few to no alternatives.

JG, CS, and TM each returned to community-specific data and coded accounts of women's experience with the cancer care system along these themes. We particularly identified moments in which low socioeconomic status, older age, or Aboriginal identity was salient to 'quality of life' – physical or emotional health going unsupported during treatment, or 'survival factors' – to assessment or treatment not received or delayed. We called these documented recollections 'moments of exclusion.' In addition to assigning themes, we were mindful about also tracking what the women did not say and who was likely to gain or lose in a given participant–healthcare professional exchange.

The Cross-community Analysis Workshop

The two-day workshop was designed to review the 'silence and voice' and 'vulnerability and resistance' findings from each project and then to attend in a deliberate way to the echoes across projects. At the workshop, we provided each individual with copies of the project-specific coded data and then asked the group to discuss whether or not these higher-level themes – silence and voice, resistance and vulnerability – were present and salient across projects. We encouraged the investigative team to engage in an iterative process of focusing upon the particularities of a woman's experience within a specific population group and then examining the same text for its similarity/dissimilarity to women's experiences in the other two project populations.

We generated the following reflections at the conclusion of the exercise:

- Silence is associated with not complaining, not asking questions of healthcare providers, and is used as a coping strategy. Silence is also associated with women's strength and independence (e.g., 'I would never ask … unless I was really desperate … I do everything I can myself.'). Silence works for and against women.
- Recode Resistance as Resilience. Resistance conjures notions of politicized action and reaction. Resilience is more about an internal and individual process and more conceptually representative of the selected quotes. The notion of resistance does, however, trigger the

reader to feel that the health system is resistant to the needs of these women.

- The health system seems designed for the 'model patient' – well educated, with access to resources, especially for recovery. Those who deviate might receive care that is inappropriate for their particular needs.
- Power of health providers within the cancer care system is perceived in specific ways (i.e., oncologist is positioned at the centre and other providers lack power).
- Women talk about their 'rights' within the health system if they've encountered rudeness, been lied to, or in particular if they viewed their experience through an anti-oppression/anti-colonial lens (which rarely occurred).

We return to many of these illuminations in the discussion and conclusion sections. Bolstered by the feedback received from the cross-analysis workshop, CS, JG, and TM wondered in what circumstances within the cancer care system do women experience these moments of exclusion? We each went back to our data, read through the circumstances of exclusion, and collapsed the data from these higher-order themes or manifestations of exclusion into three sub-themes: 'Not Getting Cancer Care,' 'Not Even Getting There,' and 'Not Getting Supportive Care.' In the interests of chapter length we will focus only on the first two sub-themes.

Findings

We identified, in these distilled themes, the ways in which the health system actively shapes marginalized women's experiences of cancer and cancer care. These experiences have been organized within two realms of exclusion: Not Getting Cancer Care and Not Even Getting There. In the Echoes across Social Locations sections we explore how health systems and health professionals organize and regulate care opportunities for marginalized women.[1]

Not Getting Cancer Care

This first realm of exclusion, Not Getting Cancer Care, focuses on not having access (including timely access) to surgery, chemotherapy, radiation, adjuvant treatment such as Tamoxifen – an adjuvant treatment medication typically prescribed to women for five years – and side effect medications (including antinauseants). Also within this category are examples of how women chose not to receive treatment in part because of worries that they would not be well supported during recovery. These stories reflect women's subjective assessments.

OLDER WOMEN

Lisa, diagnosed with breast cancer at age 81, 'refused anything to do with chemo.' She expressed some pride that she was able to take a stand against the physician's advice: 'If I hadn't given it thought well before, I might not have been strong enough to say "I don't need it."' She explained her decision this way:

> I don't think [the physician] really understood until I said 'quality of life with chemo' didn't appeal to me all. I live alone, I like it and I know many people who have gone through it and depended on whoever's handy … I know my hairdresser told me about her friend and his children abandoned him and he, of course, didn't have much to eat even. (Lisa)

Lisa perceived that the side effects of chemotherapy might jeopardize her ability to continue living at home independently. The choice she makes consciously preserves her independence and dignity; insisting on her right to make this choice, she claims voice and asserts power. At the same time, of course, Lisa's choice unfolds in a particular social context. In Ontario, worries about depending on 'whoever's handy' for care are heightened by the steady erosion of state-funded supportive home care (Aronson & Neysmith, 2001). While the choice to forgo treatment reflects strength and self-determination, it is also clear that worries about the effects of cancer treatment and their appraisals of their options are shaped by the wider political economies of care.

LOWER-INCOME WOMEN

An Ontario survey cataloguing the out-of-pocket expenses for cancer patients (n=282: 74 breast, 70 colorectal, 68 lung, 70 prostate) reported high average monthly costs for prescription drugs ($45, range $0–$1400)[2] (Longo, Deber, Fitch, & Williams, 2004). The women in the lower-income study found it difficult to pay the dispensing fees, and those who did not have private insurance or who were unaware of public insurance drug programs could not afford supportive-care drugs, such as anti-nausea pills. At the time of their treatment, four of five women from the lower-income study who were prescribed Tamoxifen were required to pay for it out of pocket. One woman noted her vulnerability when describing her lack of ability to afford treatment medications and the associated dispensing fees.

> So you're not anticipating that there's [anti-nausea] drugs out there that cost one hundred dollars a pill, you know? ... [the dispensing fee is] ten or eleven dollars depending which pharmacy you go to ... I still had to pay the dispensing fee on it ... even that can be a hardship. (Rose)

This vulnerability raises the concern that women will choose not to fill their treatment prescriptions or that they will not be able to access them in a timely way. This woman also spoke about her strategy to reduce the costs of prescribed medications.

> And [the clinical trial nurse] would be cooperative enough that she would order two prescriptions in one so that I only had to pay one dispensing fee. I mean, she was working with me the whole time with this. And you know, you say it's only ten bucks or eleven dollars, but it makes a difference. So she did do that, she got the doctors to just write the prescription for multiples in one. (Rose)

Unfortunately, Rose's strategy is dependent on the will or interest of healthcare providers to thwart the health system. Rose did not have resources to ensure that her prescriptions could be doubled-up. Her resilience demonstrates the neglect of the health system to address these particular financial needs. Fortunately for Rose, this scenario also points to penetrability of the health system by the health providers.

ABORIGINAL WOMEN

Despite the reality that Aboriginal women are at much higher risk of getting cervical cancer and have lower survival rates for all cancers (Marrett & Chaudhry, 2003), cancer information, screening, and treatment resources are not addressing this fact (Hislop et al., 1992). Michelle provided an emotionally charged story of not getting informed and timely cancer care. While cancer patients generally experience the dread of waiting for diagnoses and prognoses (the period of not knowing), this individual expresses her concern about having to wait an extended period of time before she learned about a possible treatment plan.

I fell through the cracks between my first visit with the oncologist and the surgeon. I don't know what happened, but I am waiting for the surgeon to contact me ... nobody contacted me for about four weeks. (Michelle)

Experiences such as this also interact with historical experiences of colonialism, leaving these women feeling excluded and as though their lives lack value. Michelle was simultaneously confronted by a cancer diagnosis and left to worry about the nature and scheduling of her treatment. The Native Advisory Committee of this study felt that the delays in treatment and follow-up were of grave concern as delays in diagnosis and treatment might be directly associated with poorer five-year survival outcomes (Burhansstipanov, Gilbert, LaMarca, & Krebs, 2002; Marrett & Chaudhry, 2003).

Echoes across Social Locations

Presumably, features of patient-centred care include timely and affordable treatment, the opportunity to receive that care in a respectful manner, and the offer and receipt of adequate and accessible home care services. The women in these critical examples are not receiving this care, or optimal cancer care; they are refusing treatment, experiencing delays, or taking 'risky' steps to access health resources. For example, a refusal to accept treatment could contribute to an unnecessarily decreased lifespan, and accessing doubled-up prescriptions occurs at the mercy of providers willing to bend the rules. These women all demonstrate resilience and self-determination when encountering an inadequate health system but do so at considerable cost, in ways that reflect their marginalized position and at a physically and emotionally precarious time in their lives.

Not Even Getting There

In the Ontario survey discussed above (Longo et al., 2004) patients reported mean monthly expenses of $213 when travel costs were excluded and $646 when they were included. Free transportation services are provided by the Canadian Cancer Society, but women from marginalized communities do not always know this. In the following stories, it becomes clear that if these women had known of this service, the odds of them getting to the treatment centre would increase.

OLDER WOMEN

Transportation frequently posed a problem for older study participants, echoing findings from a study by Goodwin, Hunt, and Samet
(1993) where patients who drove or who lived with a driver were four
times more likely to receive radiation. For participants in our studies,
the importance of free transportation services was apparent:[3]

LISA: I doubt I'd have had radiation if I hadn't had transportation ... I
    had no other means and there's no way I could get a bus and get up
    there. Some of the appointments were for, what, 7:30, I got up very
    early and there'd be no way that I could ...
INTERVIEWER: You were able to manage early morning appointments
    but not on your own.
LISA: But not on the bus.
INTERVIEWER: It would really be the public transportation and you're
    not driving, you don't have a car.
LISA: Oh, no! [laughter] (Lisa, diagnosed at 81)

For Lisa, transportation was available but dependent upon the generos-
ity and availability of volunteers participating in this volunteer service.
Getting women who have cancer to the health system for treatment is
not a formal part of the health system. For other participants, free services were not always accessible.

LOWER-INCOME WOMEN

Twelve of the fourteen women in the lower-income women study needed to travel to receive chemotherapy and/or radiation treatment. Many
women described paying the cancer centre parking fees as a 'hardship.'
Five of these twelve women requiring transportation reported driving
to the cancer treatment centre and, for several reasons, were uncon-
cerned about parking expenses. One of these five women knew of and
used a free transportation service provided by a local cancer organization. Of the remaining seven women, two women walked to and from
treatments, three used public transit, one had friends drop her off and
pick her up, and one women took a state-funded taxi until she could no
longer afford to pre-pay for this service (a requirement of participating
in a social assistance or welfare program). Deanna struggles between
feeling empowered to make a positive budgeting choice to forgo treatment appointments against realizing that her good money managing
skills are borne of necessity and the lack of choice.

I consider myself pretty good on budgeting my money. But at the same time I've had to live on five hundred bucks a month for the last, I don't know how many years you know, and you learn that you don't have a choice but to do that ... So now this [transportation to Hospital 1] is like a big expense [it is] a problem cause there's days I don't have the money ... one week I had a bone scan one day, the next day I had some other tests, then I had another test the third day and chemo ... I [would] phone and say I'm sorry but, it's not like I don't want to come but ... I was only getting five hundred [a month] at the time [from a provincial income security program] ... I go to [the cancer treatment centre] it's ten dollars there, ten dollars back. If I go three times a week there's sixty dollars, four times sixty is two hundred and forty dollars. (Deanna)

ABORIGINAL WOMEN

Aboriginal communities are often rural and remote. Geographic and cultural location means that many of these communities are among the medically unserved and underserved populations in Canada (Adelson, 2005; Stout, Kipling, & Stout, 2001; Till, 2003). During the interviews, Aboriginal participants relayed that transportation to treatment centres and telephone bills during treatment were a drain on individual and family resources. They were not necessarily identified as social problems, however – rather as ways of life.

There is a family doctor who flies to the community about once a month or so. If I want to or have to see a specialist there is one who comes to the community about every six months. Or if there is such a doctor visiting Iqaluit which is about 200 miles south west of [my community], then I would have to fly to see them ...

My biggest problem was, where am I going to stay while I'm in treatment. I'm in [name of a large city] for treatment which is about 3000 miles from home. (Lynea)

Lynea's cancer story is a powerful story of limited access; the burden of cancer magnified by infrequent contact with physicians, not to mention specialists such as oncologists. She tells of the difficulty of finding accommodation when so far from her home and community. Although Lynea is a member of a vulnerable population, she considers our research questions about her vulnerability as a Native woman to be racist. She mentions to the interviewer that she is strong, resilient, and actively resists racism. However, her access to screening and care is nevertheless characterized and limited by geographic and systemic barriers.

Echoes across Social Locations

The cancer system is organized for people with private transportation who can pay to park week after week and weeks at a time at cancer centres or hospitals. Accessibility to cancer care is compromised for people who are not in a stable financial position. We discovered that treatment 'choices' are determined by finances and that women will even 'choose' to drop out of or modify treatments when they cannot transport themselves to the cancer centre, manage treatment effects, or maintain their roles in the family or workplace. We do not know how or whether missing treatment contributes to lower survival rates among these populations. So far, these research studies have not been designed and implemented. However, this construal of patient 'choice' is troubling. It draws our attention to the ways that social location shapes access to quality of cancer care.

Discussion

Our intentions for this research were to:

1 Explore the meanings and everyday life experiences behind the labels Aboriginal women with cancer, older women with cancer, and low-income women with cancer.
2 Share tools and substantive knowledge about the processes – both community-specific and common among communities of women – that link poverty, Aboriginal identity, and older age to quality of life and possibly survival in the current healthcare context.

We derived the following learning from this cross-analysis process:

• It is possible to analyse across diverse sets of data if the focus of these efforts is to understand parallel, and not necessarily identical, experience. For example, we needed to examine parallel but not identical instances of the process of exclusion.
• Cross-analysis was made manageable when we chose to scrutinize parallel experiences at particular junctures in the cancer trajectory such as 'getting there' and 'getting cancer care.'

- Having the individual project analysis already completed for the two-day workshop and the prepartory work for the cross-analysis underway (i.e., identifying the themes for discussion – silence and voice, vulnerability and resistence) was found by the participants to be an efficient way to work.
- Working with a multi-discipline team provided fertile ground for richer discussion than could have been accomplished among the lead investigators only.

These tools, and the development of them, helped us get behind the meanings in notions of silence and voice, vulnerability and resilience, and to disorganize and to disorient those meanings. In so doing, we were able to identify health system accountability. In short, the findings presented in this chapter suggest that Aboriginal, low-income, and older women experience similar forms of marginalization across social locations, marginalization which is exacerbated by cancer care systems.

The Cancer System and Exclusion

It appears from the data presented here that women from marginalized social locations do not always receive and/or perceive optimal cancer care and treatment. These reported circumstances affect their quality of life and might affect their survival. Individual narrative accounts of personal resilience, such as missing a treatment or deciding to forgo chemotherapy in order to manage finances or retain independence, ultimately reveal barriers to optimal care and unmask the otherwise invisible responsibility of the health system to provide effective cancer treatment to a variety of cancer patients.

Viewing the data through feminist lenses we can understand the inequities experienced by women across social locations in a particular way. These moments of exclusion are embedded in power relations with those who set up services or even with individual health professionals in the health system, and they manifest or echo across social locations. Weber and Parra-Medina (2003) explain,

> because feminist scholarship conceives of race, class, gender ... as social constructions that are generated, challenged, and maintained in group processes, the place to observe and thus to understand inequality is in dynamic interactions among groups, particularly among those that involve groups experiencing multiple oppressions. (p. 203)

By regarding the echoes of experience retold here as social construc-
tions, we can view the ways in which women were at an advantage
or disadvantage, had options or did not have options as members of
non-dominant or marginalized social groups when seeking cancer care.

Currently the Ontario cancer care system, despite claims to patient-
centredness, appears premised on a model patient – a patient who is
part of the dominant social group, with all attendant resources and
privileges (Sherwin, 1998). Research with lesbians with cancer (Sinding, Barnoff, & Grassau, 2004) and low-income women with cancer
(Gould, 2004) lends strength to this finding. The ways current services
reflect the meanings of dominant groups and premise themselves on
economic resources are pressing issues in the social science study of
illness (Sinding & Wiernikowski, 2008). Not fitting the ideal for the
model patient can translate into less than optimal or ill-fitting healthcare services for marginalized communities of women. 'Not getting'
resources from within the cancer system might tell us as much about
systemic dysfunction as it does about social vulnerability. Unfortunately, health professionals lack satisfactory frameworks or protocols
to serve the needs of cancer patients that do not fit the 'ideal' or 'model
patient.'

Clinical or Policy Implications

This study underscores the ways that the broader structures of oppression are expressed through and are accorded power in the policies and
practices of the cancer care system, and how they worsen the experience
of marginalization for women who are poor, Aboriginal, and older. Any
one form of marginalization might also include compounding barriers
of social exclusion, as well as cultural, linguistic, and geographic barriers to cancer care.

Despite public funding of hospital and physician services across Canada, marginalized women's stories provide evidence of how embedded
inequalities within the health system shape differential access to cancer
care. Further, though provincial governments have withdrawn resources from the health system, these resources have not been reallocated to
address social determinants of health – and so, marginalized women
experience the withdrawal of resources or the lack of access to them,
which exacerbates already difficult social conditions.

We note that the lack of access to health services is a disputed social determinant of health. For example, although low socioeconomic status is associated with poor health outcomes in most illnesses, some authors believe that poor health in individuals who experience this disadvantage is more likely due to 'unfavorable social conditions and ineffective self-management than from limitations in access to care' (Pincus, Esther, DeWalt, & Callahan, 1998, p. 407). These same authors propose that social policy focus on education, resources to elevate social conditions, and research on self-management. Raphael (2003) argues against the focus on lifestyle risk factors by citing that these factors 'account for only a small proportion of variation in incidence among individuals in heart disease, cancers and diabetes' (p. 35). Were a country to focus on national strategies to mitigate the ill-effects associated with social determinants of health, such as pouring money and resources into promoting social capital, improving working conditions, and encouraging healthy lifestyles as have been implemented in Sweden, then we would advance the goal to eradicate social ills (Raphael).

Even if health services are not considered to be a *fundamental* cause of health disparities, we argue that in the cancer field, health system inequalities both contribute to – and can mitigate – broader inequities.

To begin to agitate for an equitable shift in the cancer care system we ask the following questions:

- How can full access to cancer treatment and supportive care be ensured for all cancer patients and not just the model patients?
- What is the responsibility of the Canadian health system and professional regulatory bodies to transform the social practices and relations that institutionalize exclusion (Gustafson, 2005)?
- How can community-based care systems such as home care, community transportation services for those with cancer, and support services offered by community agencies become more available and equitable?

Limitations of the Research

We have described experiences of exclusion across populations of marginalized women. We did not, however, address the complex identities of individual women. For example, a few Aboriginal women interviewed for this research were also living in lower-income circumstances, as were many older women. Among participants in the low-income study were women of colour. The social locations of women who participated in the research varied beyond the three identity categories explored for the purposes of this project. The effort to make claims for particular women within particular social locations has obvious limitations.

Conclusion

Understanding the full implications of social location is problematic. But, we have resolved that as a first step it is important to give voice to communities of marginalized women whose exclusion stories are otherwise not contained in the cancer literature in so far as those relayed experiences provide insight into their quality of cancer care and possible threats to their survival. We cannot expect that already marginalized individuals will feel free to criticize the health system in a time of health crisis. This study was strengthened, then, by its commitment to listen to three communities of women. Voices from three communities, coming together, strengthen the call for change.

Women from marginalized communities may not receive the care they need because the health system is designed to respond to 'model patients.' Health professionals miss stories of suboptimal care both because they are ill-prepared to respond to other than the model patient and because women's claims are muted. This mismatch between health systems organized around a model patient and individual, marginalized women (coping with a racist, classist, sexist, ageist society) renders health professionals unable to consistently assist these women in effective ways. We need to think about and to question a health system that is organized around the model patient with the goal of sparing marginalized women the task of negotiating with a cancer system while negotiating cancer.

Acknowledgments

Many thanks to the women who participated in each of the three projects (Older Women, Aboriginal Women, and Lower-Income Women studies). The Intersecting Vulnerabilities research program was funded by the Canadian Institutes of Health Research. The Older Women Study was also supported by a grant from McMaster University. The Canadian Breast Cancer Foundation, Ontario Chapter funds the Ontario Breast Cancer Community Research Initiative, home of the Intersecting Vulnerabilities research program.

NOTES

This chapter is based on Gould et al. (in press): 'Below their notice': Exploring women's subjective experiences of cancer system exclusion.

1 Please note all names documented below are pseudonyms.
2 The data are skewed by the small number of patients who reported out-of-pocket expenses. For example, only 39 of 277 reported any costs for assistive devices, but those who did often paid significant amounts.
3 Transportation services such as those provided by the Canadian Cancer Society, a national community-based organization of volunteers, whose mission includes the enhancement of the quality of life of people living with cancer.

REFERENCES

Adelson, N. (2005). The embodiment of inequity: Health disparities in Aboriginal Canada. *Canadian Journal of Public Health, 96*(2), S45–61.
Aronson, J., & Neysmith, S. (2001). Manufacturing social exclusion in the home care market. *Canadian Public Policy, 27*(2), 151–65.
Balducci, L. (2001). The geriatric cancer patient: Equal benefit from equal treatment. *Cancer Control, 8*(2, Suppl.), 1–25.
Baum, F. (1995). Researching public health: Behind the qualitative-quantitative methodological debate. *Social Science and Medicine, 40,* 459–68.
Burhansstipanov, L. (2001). Cancer: A growing problem among American Indians and Alaska Natives. In M. Dixon and Y. Roubideaux (Eds.), *Promises to Keep* (chap. 10). Washington: American Public Health Association.
Burhansstipanov, L., Gilbert, A., LaMarca, K., & Krebs, L.U. (2002). An innovative path to improving cancer care in Indian Country. *Public Health Reports, 116,* 424–33.
Canada. Federal, Provincial and Territorial Advisory Committee on Population Health. (1996). *Report on the health of Canadians.* Ottawa: Minister of Supply and Services Canada.
Canada. Health Canada. (1999). The health of senior women. Ottawa: Department of Health. Available at http://www.hc-sc.gc.ca/hl-vs/pubs/women-femmes/index-eng.php
Canadian Cancer Society/ National Cancer Institute of Canada. (2007). *Canadian cancer statistics 2007.* Toronto, Canada.
Crooks, D.L. (2001). Older women with breast cancer: New understandings

through grounded theory research. *Health Care Women International, 22*(1–2), 99–114.

Davis, T., Williams, M., Marin, E., Parker, R., & Glass, J. (2002). Health literacy and cancer communication. *CA: A Cancer Journal for Clinicians, 52,* 134–49.

Eyles, J., Birch, S., & Newbold, K.B. (1995). Delivering the goods? Access to family physician services in Canada: A comparison of 1985 and 1991. *Journal of Health and Social Behavior, 36,* 322–32.

Farley, T.A., & Flannery, J.T. (1989). Late stages diagnosis of breast cancer in women of lower income socioeconomic status: Public health implications. *American Journal of Public Health, 79*(11), 1508–12.

Goodwin, J.S., Hunt, W.C., & Samet, J.M. (1993). Determinants of cancer therapy in elderly patients. *Cancer, 72,* 594–601.

Gould, J. (2004). Lower-income women with breast cancer: Interacting with cancer treatment and income security systems. *Canadian Woman Studies, 24*(1), 31–6.

Gould, J., Sinding, C., Mitchell, T., Gustafson, D., Peng, I., McGillicuddy, P., Fitch, M., Aronson, J. (in press). 'Below their notice': Exploring women's subjective experiences of cancer system exclusion. *Journal of Cancer Education.*

Gray, R., Goel, V., Fitch, M., Franssen, E., Chart, P., Greenberg, M., et al. (2000). Utilization of professional supportive care services by women with breast cancer. *Breast Cancer Research and Treatment, 64,* 253–8.

Guadagnoli, E., Shapiro, C., Gurwitz, J.H., Silliman, R.A., Weeks, J.C., Borbas, C., et al. (1997). Age-related patterns of care: Evidence against ageism in the treatment of early-stage breast cancer. *Journal of Clinical Oncology, 15,* 2338–44.

Gustafson, D.L. (2005). Transcultural nursing theory from a critical cultural perspective. *Advances in Nursing Science, 28*(1), 2–16.

Hislop, T.G., Deschamps, M., Band, P.R., Smith, J.M., & Clarke, H.F. (1992). Participation in the British Columbia Cervical Cytology Screening Programme by Native Indian women. *Canadian Journal Public Health, 83,* 344–5.

Kagawa-Singer, M., & Kassim-Lakha, S. (2003). A strategy to reduce cross-cultural miscommunication and increase the likelihood of improving health outcomes. *Academic Medicine: Journal of the Association of American Medical Colleges, 78,* 577–87.

Karjalainen, S., & Pukkala, E. (1990). Social class as a prognostic factor in breast cancer survival. *Cancer, 66,* 819–27.

Kasper, A. (2002) Barriers and burdens: Poor women face breast cancer. In A. Kasper & S. Ferguson (Eds.), *Breast cancer: Society shapes an epidemic*. New York: St Martin's Press.

Kearney, N., & Miller, M. (2000). Elderly patients with cancer: An ethical dilemma. *Critical Reviews in Oncology Hematology, 33*(2), 149–54.

Lannin, D.R., Mathews, H.F., Mitchell, J., Swanson, M.S., Swanson, F.H., & Edwards, M.S. (1998). Influence of socioeconomic and cultural factors on racial differences in late-stage presentation of breast cancer. *Journal of the American Medical Association, 279,* 1801–7.

Lantz, P.M., Orians, C.E., Liebow, E., Burhansstipanov, L., Erb, J., & Kenyon, K. (2003). Implementing women's cancer screening programs in American Indian and Alaska Native populations. *Health Care for Women International, 24,* 674–96.

Lickley, H.L. (1997). Primary breast cancer in the elderly. *Canadian Journal of Surgery, 40,* 341–51.

Longo, C., Deber, R., Fitch, M., & Williams, A. (2004). Characteristics of out-of-pocket costs for cancer patients in Ontario, Canada. *Journal of Clinical Oncology, ASCO Annual Meeting Proceedings (Post-Meeting Edition), 22*(14S) (July 15 Suppl.), 8251.

Macintyre, S. (1986). The patterning of health by social position in contemporary Britain: Directions for sociological research. *Social Science and Medicine, 23,* 393–415.

Mackillop, W.J., Zhang-Salomons, J., Groome, P.A., Paszat, L., & Holowaty, E. (1997). Socioeconomic status and cancer survival in Ontario. *Journal of Clinical Oncology, 15,* 1680–9.

Macleod, U., Ross, S., Gillis, C., McConnachie, A., Twelves, C., & Watt, C. (2000). Socio-economic deprivation and stage of disease at presentation in women with breast cancer. *Annals of Oncology, 11,* 105–7.

MacMillan, H.L., MacMillan, A.B., Offord, D.R., & Dingle, J.L. (1996). Aboriginal health. *Canadian Medical Association Journal, 155,* 1569–78.

Marrett, L.D., & Chaudhry, M. (2003). Cancer incidence and mortality in Ontario First Nations, 1968–1991 (Canada). *Cancer Causes and Control, 14*(3), 259–68.

McDonald, I., & Daly, J. (1992). Researching methods in health care: Summing up. In D.J. McDonald & E. Willis (Eds.), *Researching health care: Designs, dilemmas, disciplines*. London: Routledge.

Minkler, M., & Wallerstein, N. (Eds.). (2003). *Community-based participatory research for health*. San Francisco: Jossey-Bass.

Mitchell, T., & Baker, E. (2005). Community building vs career building research. The challenges, risks, and responsibilities of conducting participatory cancer research with Aboriginal communities. *Journal of Cancer Education*, *20*, 41–6.

Mitchell, T., & St. Germaine-Small, M. (2005). *The silence that surrounds Aboriginal women with breast or cervical cancer*. Unpublished manuscript.

Moore, K. (1999). Breast cancer patients' out-of-pocket expenses. *Oncology Nursing Forum*, *22*, 389–96.

Morse, J.M. (1995). Exploring the theoretical basis of nursing using advanced techniques of concept analysis. *Advances in Nursing Science*, *17*(3), 31–46.

Muss, H. (2002). *Breast cancer in older women*. Paper presented at the ASCO Educational Symposium: Cancer Care in the Older Population.

Ontario. Cancer Care Ontario. (2002). 'It's our responsibility…': Aboriginal cancer care needs assessment report. Toronto.

Ontario Community Support Association. (2001). In 20 short years: A discussion paper on demographics and aging. Retrieved August 10, 2007, from http://www.ocsa.on.ca/PDF/In_20_Short_Years.PDF

Patton, M.A. (2001). *Qualitative research and evaluation methods* (3rd ed.). Thousand Oaks, CA: Sage Publications.

Pincus, T., Esther, R., DeWalt, D., & Callahan, F. (1998). Social conditions and self-management are more powerful determinants of health than access to care. *Annals of Internal Medicine*, *129*, 406–11.

Raphael, D. (2003). Addressing the social determinants of health in Canada: Bridging the gap between research findings and public policy. *Policy Options*, March, 35–40.

Sherwin, S. (1998). A relational approach to autonomy in health care. In S. Sherwin (Ed.), *The Politics of Women's Health* (pp. 19–47). Philadelphia: Temple University Press.

Silliman, R.A. (2003). What constitutes optimal care for older women with breast cancer? *Journal of Clinical Oncology*, *21*, 3554–6.

Silliman, R.A., Troyan, S.L., Guadagnoli, E., Kaplan, S.H., & Greenfield, S. (1997). The impact of age, marital status, and physician-patient interactions on the care of older women with breast carcinoma. *Cancer*, *80*, 1326–34.

Siminoff, L.A., Zhang, A., Saunders Sturm, C.M., & Colabianchi, N. (2000). Referral of breast cancer patients to medical oncologists after initial surgical management. *MedCare*, *38*, 696–704.

Sinding, C., Barnoff, L., & Grassau, P. (2004). Homophobia and heterosexism in cancer care: Lesbians' experiences. *Canadian Journal of Nursing Research*, *36*, 170–88.

Sinding, C., & Wiernikowski, J. (2008). Disruption foreclosed: Older women's cancer narratives. *Health: An Interdisciplinary Journal for the Social Study of Health, Illness & Medicine, 12*(3), 389–411.

Sinding, C., Wiernikowski, J., & Aronson, J. (2005). Cancer care from the perspectives of older women. *Oncology Nursing Forum, 32,* 1169–75.

Stout, M.D., Kipling, G.D., & Stout, R. (2001). Aboriginal women's health research synthesis project: Final report. Centres of Excellence for Women's Health Program, Women's Health Bureau, Health Canada. Retrieved May 25, 2005, from www.cwhn.ca/resources/synthesis/synthesis-en.pdf

Till, J.E. (2003). Evaluation of support groups for women with breast cancer: Importance of the navigator role. *Health and Quality of Life Outcomes, 1,* 16.

Turner, N.J., Haward, R.A., Mulley, G.P., & Selby, P.J. (1999). Cancer in old age – is it inadequately investigated and treated? *British Medical Journal, 319,* 309–12.

Wanebo, H.J., Cole, B., Chung, M., Vezeridis, M., Schepps, B., Fulton, J., et al. (1997). Is surgical management compromised in elderly patients with breast cancer? *Annals of Surgery, 225,* 579–86.

Wang, L., & Arnold, K. (2002). Low socioeconomic status may influence quality of breast cancer treatment. *Journal of the National Cancer Institute, 94,* 467.

Watters, J.M., Yau, J.C., O'Rourke, K., Tomiak, E., & Gertler, S.Z. (2003). Functional status is well maintained in older women during adjuvant chemotherapy for breast cancer. *Annals of Oncology, 14*(12), 1744–50.

Weber, L., & Parra-Medina, S. (2003). Intersectionality and women's health: Charting a path to eliminating health disparities. Gender perspectives on health and medicine: Key themes. *Advances in Gender Research, 7,* 181–230.

Yancik, R., Wesley, M.N., Ries, L.A., Havlik, R.J., Edwards, B.K., & Yates, J.W. (2001). Effect of age and comorbidity in postmenopausal breast cancer patients aged 55 years and older. *Journal of the American Medical Association, 285,* 885–92.

Yarborough, S. (2004). Older women and breast cancer screening: Research synthesis. *Oncology Nursing Forum, 31*(1), 9–15.

5 'Nurses Can't Do It. They Have a Hundred and Ten Patients': Health Professionals' Working Conditions and the Experiences of Informal Caregivers

CHRIS SINDING

The majority of deaths in Canada occur in hospitals (Heyland, Lavery, Tranmer, Shortt, & Taylor, 2000). Yet most of dying takes place at home (Rhodes & Shaw, 1999), and most care for people who are dying is provided informally by family members and friends.

Trends supporting home-based provision of palliative care reflect shifts in the wider economic and political context of healthcare provision. Since the mid-1970s, public discourse and government policy (prompted by economic globalization – see Coburn, 1999) has organized a relatively residual role for the state in the care of people who are disabled, elderly, or ill. Congruent with neo-liberal principles, the market has assumed greater importance in the allocation and distribution of care. Informal social networks, as well, have a much more critical (even celebrated) role.

The research I describe here explored people's accounts of caring for a relative or friend who died of breast cancer. I was drawn to this research in part through my relationship with Jan Livingston, who had been a driving force in an OBCCRI project. Jan was part of the team that developed and toured the drama *Handle with Care? Women Living with Metastastic Breast Cancer.* Jan was a marvellously feisty and funny woman, utterly passionate about the work we were doing to give voice and visibility to the experiences of women like her, living with advanced cancer. As Jan was dying, I was struck by the grace and tenacity her daughter and friends exhibited and the struggle they experienced. I was also struck by health professionals' roles in all this. In my research, I wanted to explore how the experience of caring for someone who is dying is made more difficult, and how it is eased, by meanings drawn from interactions with professionals.

Table 6

INFORMAL PALLIATIVE CARE

Why was the research completed?
This research explored people's stories of caring for a relative or friend who died of breast cancer. I was drawn to the study in part through my relationship with Jan Livingston, who played a key role in another OBCCRI project. As Jan was dying, her daughters and friends showed incredible grace and tenacity, and they struggled. In Canada, most care for people who are dying is provided by family members and friends, yet we know relatively little about their experiences and perspectives. Informal end-of-life caregiving will become even more important in the coming years, as trends supporting home-based provision of care reflect shifts in the wider economic and political context of healthcare.

What methods were used?
Two interviews were conducted with each of twelve study participants, and one carer responded by letter to a series of questions drawn from the interview guide. Among the participants were seven spouses (five husbands, one lesbian partner, and one wife), two sisters, three friends, and one daughter. Accounts were analysed with reference to grounded theory methods.

What were the key findings?
Over the course of the study, health professionals' (over)work emerged as a key link between broad trends in the health system, and the actions, experiences, and narratives of informal carers. Health policy and politics became meaningful in the lives of informal carers through their awareness of health professional strain and overwork.

What are some implications or results of the research?
In this study, caregivers' actions appeared to prompt health professionals' responsiveness to the ill person; such responsiveness may thus be unequally distributed, accruing more readily to people with strong and well-resourced kin and friendship networks. Further research is required to confirm and extend this finding, and to critically consider its implications for equity in cancer care.

As well, when family members and friends of ill people see health professionals doing the best they can in difficult circumstances, they may swallow their concerns about care. While improved strategies for

gathering care evaluations may be required, evaluation research is, in
general terms, devoid of concern with wider systemic and structural
issues. It is only in more collectively oriented social action that higher
standards of care can be established (or reestablished) as within the
purview of health professionals' duties, and thus confirmed as patients'
and carers' entitlements.

In this chapter I describe some of the messy stumbling around of
analysis, the halting process of trying to figure out what, exactly, I was
doing with interview transcripts, with all of these wrenching/thought-
ful/bitter/heartbreaking/mundane/perplexed/longing/wise-words-
on-pages. I knew that I wanted to use grounded theory methods to
analyse the interviews, but I had no idea what it meant to do this, exactly. Grounded theory calls for open and focused coding, constant
comparison within and between accounts, attention to the conditions
under which phenomena arise and the consequences associated with
the phenomena, and the use of memos to capture insights emerging
from coding (Charmaz, 1990; Strauss & Corbin, 1990; Glaser, 2004). In
this chapter, following Orono (1990) I attempt to reveal how grounded
theory methods unfolded in this particular research project. I offer examples of coding and comparison processes, describe my use of memos, and outline points of difficulty I encountered with grounded theory
methods around the 'account context' of my coding efforts. My aim
is to make visible how two approaches to the same data, both using
grounded theory methods, led to two distinct analyses.

Analytic Process

Coding

Following the conventions of grounded theory methods, I began coding interview transcripts as soon as possible after the interviews. As I
moved through sections of respondents' narratives I tried out the questions Lofland and Lofland (1995, p. 186) suggest and have compiled
from various qualitative research texts. They encourage asking, for instance, 'What can we think of this as being about?'; from Strauss and
Corbin (1990, p. 63) they draw the questions, 'What is this? What does
it represent?'; from Charmaz (1983, pp. 112, 113), 'What do I see going

on here? What are these people doing? What is happening?' The word or set of words applied to the item of data in answering such questions is, say Lofland and Lofland, a code, the basic unit of a grounded theory.

A central goal of my research – to explain how the experience of caring for a dying friend or relative is shaped by meanings drawn from interactions with health professionals – quickly found its way into the coding scheme as 'Impact Health Professional on Carer.' Yet by the third interview, it was clear that this code was not appearing with any particular frequency, and, even in places where the code seemed to fit, I felt as if I was missing something. I was also hearing and – in grounded theory fashion – working to hear echoes within and between the early transcripts of themes and topics. Talk about 'knowing' recurred. 'They wouldn't have known her in the same way,' a woman said to explain the relatively indifferent care her sister received on a new ward. I applied the code 'Knowing' without having any particular sense of how it might fit with anything else.

In carefully rereading the transcript of the second interview I was struck by the respondent's description of the 'fuss' made by the nurses over her sister, Linda, the enthusiastic commentary they offered on her hair and her clothes. When I asked Carol to say what she thought this interaction had meant to Linda, Carol spoke about how the nurses' talk gave her sister a sense of being in a social situation, among friends, and thus eased her anxiety and dread about her diagnosis. Carol's comments, then, lent some substance to my notion that health professionals' words and actions may be especially meaningful at end-of-life to ill people and their carers. Yet Carol went on to draw a parallel between what she witnessed and her own interactions with health professionals:

> I think [what the nurses said and did] meant the world to Linda. And I can certainly say just as an aside from my own experience when I was going
> · through chemo, it was colossally important. *But I made it happen*, because I would go dressed, so that they did notice me. And maybe she in her own way was doing that too.

Strauss and Corbin (1990) note that it is through the first stage of coding that one's own and others' assumptions about a phenomenon may be questioned. An assumption in my thesis proposal, unstated at the time, was that the salient effect of interactions between health professionals and carers was unidirectional and initiated by health professionals:

health professionals' words and actions affected carers. In this passage, Carol makes clear that she saw herself, and perhaps also the ill woman, taking deliberate action to affect health professionals, to be recognized and remembered – to be known in some way – by them.

I was reminded, while thinking about this passage, of a friend who makes a point of taking a briefcase to appointments with physicians. The briefcase may be empty of paper but it is full with symbolism, a deliberate attempt to gain a certain kind of recognition from health professionals. This reading and reflecting focused my attention in a different way on the passages I had labelled 'Knowing,' and I recoded several as 'Being and Becoming Known to Health Professionals.' While I did not abandon my interest in the ways carers are affected by health professionals, I did release my hold on the assumption, which had informed my thesis proposal, that health professionals were the more active agents in the interactions I was exploring.

I started to think more about how caregivers and patients perceive their own words and actions affecting health professionals and to watch for this in interviews and transcripts. In raising codes to concepts, proponents of grounded theory call for attention to the conditions under which a phenomena arises and a description of the consequences associated with the phenomena (Charmaz, 1990). In the interviews and coding that followed, then, I focused both on what prompted respondents' efforts to affect health professionals, and on how they perceived the outcomes of their actions. When I came across relevant passages of text, I explored the surrounding text – sometimes as far back as the beginning of the interview, or as far forward as the last lines – to try to see what respondents saw, what motivated them to take the action they did. I also tried to sort through what they thought they 'got' from their actions, as in what they saw happening to them and the ill person as a result of what they did or said.

In the fourth interview, Martin described his role in his wife's care through a series of analogies to his professional life. He described his role in the hospital as 'progress chasing.' I told him that 'progress chasing' was a new term for me. He explained:

Progress chasing is, you know, we got this to do next, OK, well, is it happening? ... I used to do this with suppliers, I'd say, well, I know my suppliers are not going to call me with a quotation. They're just not going to do it. Well, how am I going to get it? I got to ring them. I expect to ring them. I expect to do half their job.

'Progress chasing' provided a neat *in vivo* category to link all kinds of things informal carers did: reporting instances of the ill person's discomfort, monitoring the ill person's care needs, tracking down nurses to provide care. More importantly, however, the notion of progress chasing (particularly how Martin explained it) led me to wonder about the ways informal carers' expectations of health professionals might be a condition of informal carers' actions – specifically their expectations about the extent to which nurses and doctors can be relied upon to 'do their jobs.'

The first woman I interviewed had spoken at length about the difficult work circumstances she saw community nurses facing. While I had coded this, I had not thought it particularly important. I returned to this section to see if I could discern a pathway between her comment on health professionals' working conditions and her own actions. I continued to interview, and as I worked with the transcripts I began drawing diagrams that traced each carer's actions from conditions (including perceptions of strain and overwork among health professionals) to actions (including progress chasing) to outcomes (including, for example, more timely care). It was through this process – which in its reporting here has a clear and sequential quality quite absent from its doing! – that an analysis emerged of the connections between the conditions of health professionals' work and the actions of informal carers (see the section below titled Perceptions of Health Professionals' Working Conditions: Effects on Informal Carers' Actions).

Memos

I came to this research with an interest in the interface between formal and informal palliative care. Empirical studies focused on informal carers in their relationship to formal palliative care services are generally conceptualized in terms of carer satisfaction (Fakhoury, McCarthy, & Addington-Hall, 1996a, 1996b; Jarrett, Payne, & Wiles, 1999; Kristjanson, 1986, 1989; Kristjanson, Leis, Koop, Carriere, & Mueller, 1997; Kristjanson, Sloan, Dudgeon, & Adaskin, 1996; Payne, Smith, & Dean, 1999; Seale, 1992; Skorupka & Bohnet, 1982). While my concerns in this area were defined in broader terms I was nevertheless alert, from my exploration of the literature, to study respondents' accounts of (dis)satisfaction with care. I developed codes to mark difficult healthcare experiences and experiences that were supportive, along with codes to mark both critical and laudatory commentary on care.

As I continued to code I used the qualitative analysis software NVivo to print compilations of the sections of text marked by the same code. This allowed easy comparison between all of the 'positive health care experiences' and 'difficult health care experiences' and all of text reflecting positive and negative evaluations of care. I created memos to record the questions and puzzles that emerged as I reviewed these reports. In one memo, I wrote:

> Experiences of suffering are not always associated with expressions of dissatisfaction (with health professionals or health care). Sometimes people speak praise when they or the cared-for person had discomfort / suffering, even when health professionals clearly implicated. Complaints seem to lose steam – get withdrawn?

Attempting to articulate what I saw 'going on' in study respondents' accounts, I spent considerable time working up metaphors, using memos to explore terms and images that might capture analytic insights. I also spent time rifling through my thesaurus, and wishing I had done more crossword puzzles. The search for words that addressed the many dimensions of what was happening with respondents' assessments of care – and also linked those dimensions – was, for me, an extremely useful analytic exercise, confirming Coffey and Atkinson's (1996) contention that metaphors (and figurative language more broadly) can be fruitfully employed as part of the process of data analysis.

I worked for a while with the idea that respondents' complaints about health professionals and health services were 'palliated' in the course of talk. The metaphor of palliation had obvious appeal, linked as it was to the substantive area I was exploring. It also usefully evoked two key aspects of what I saw happening with expressions of dissatisfaction: in the course of the narrative, the pain of the story was both eased and covered up. Yet as I drew and redrew diagrams that started from an account of a difficult experience, and plotted how that experience was discussed over the course of the transcript, the metaphor of 'disarmed' seemed to more thoroughly connote the range of 'what was going on' with respondents' complaints.

Defining Account Contexts

As my file of coded transcripts grew wider I started to feel as though something was not quite working. The questions I was asking the data started to feel inadequate, as if they were not moving me forward. For example, I was using the code 'Accounting for Health Professionals.' Yet this code did not seem to be organizing the data in a way that facilitated any particularly fruitful analysis. I remember thinking, with some frustration, that any particular passage of text could reasonably be 'about' at least a dozen different things within the domain of my research focus. In the file of memos where I tracked things methodological, I wrote: 'Accounting for health professionals *how*? Accounting for health professionals *why*? Accounting for health professionals *in relation to what*?'

Having reached this stage, I reviewed my memos and created a list of topics that I wanted to 'say something about' in my thesis. For instance, I wanted to discuss the responsibilities informal carers assumed. I also wanted to talk about the apparent mismatch between their (difficult) experiences and their (positive) assessments of health professionals. I began to ask in coding, 'what do I see going on here, *in relation to carers' responsibilities*?' 'what do I see going on here, *in relation to satisfaction with care*?'

At this point my coding and memo-writing became much more analytically productive. And yet something still felt discordant. The answers to questions I posed to the text felt as though they belonged in different categories; they had an 'apples and oranges' quality. I eventually realized that I was answering, and thus coding, in relation to two different contexts. Sometimes when I asked, 'what do I see going on here?' I would answer (that is, code the text) in terms of what was 'going on' in the action of caregiving. At other times, I would answer in terms of what was 'going on' in respondents' talk about caregiving. For example: in the narratives I gathered, comments about health professionals' difficult working conditions, particularly about how busy nurses are, were common, and associated with diminished expectations of professionals. In relation to the action of caregiving, I coded these comments 'Releasing Health Professionals' to signal that carers, aware that nurses and doctors were overburdened, sometimes released or excused them from responsibility for regular care duties. The same text, in the context of 'satisfaction talk,' was coded 'Disarmed Complaint,' to indicate how awareness of health professionals' difficult working conditions served to mollify or short-circuit carers' expressions of dissatisfaction with care.

As I became more aware of slipping between the two contexts I tried to reorient my coding practices, to code more systematically in relation to what was happening in the action of caregiving. Yet over time I continued to be engaged by both account contexts, and my analysis eventually proceeded in parallel lines. In one paper written from this study, talk is taken as relatively transparent, with lived experience as the subject of inquiry; respondents' experiences of providing care as the experiences happened, in the time frame of the ill person's dying, are the focus. In another paper talk itself is the subject, with attention directed to how respondents speak about difficult healthcare experiences months or years after they take place.

The Final Analyses ...

So, having followed two analytic pathways, where did I arrive? At two different destinations ... two distinct analyses with a common theme: the awareness on the part of family members and friends that nurses and physicians have 'so much to do and [there are] so few of them.' Over the course of caregiving, this perception of health professionals as overworked led family members and friends to take on care responsibilities and to devise ways to secure care from professionals. In their talk about caregiving, the perception of health professionals' overwork 'disarmed' informal carers' complaints about inadequate care.

Perceptions of Health Professionals' Working Conditions:
Effects on Informal Carers' Actions

In her narrative about caring for her partner, Ellen described arriving at the hospital at seven o'clock each morning to provide practical care: helping Jill on the commode, getting basins so she could brush her teeth and wash her face. Ellen did not suggest that Jill would not have had these basic needs met had Ellen not been there; just that she would have had to wait. In this regard Ellen describes watching as the other women in Jill's hospital room rang for a nurse and then waited:

> In the morning they're just so busy doing things, the nurses ... One woman sat on the edge of the bed and she'd just wait. She'd just sit waiting for someone to come and I really believe it's because they don't have the staff ... If they had to go to the bathroom – and these are cancer patients, these are people that maybe they can't hold it you know that sort of ... I mean Jill wouldn't have been able to wait.

Obviously the perception that health professionals were overworked was not the only reason family members and friends provided the care that they did. Ellen herself saw her decision to ensure that Jill did not wait partly in the category of 'catering' to Jill's 'whims,' 'mothering her to pieces.' Yet as is clear from this quote, Ellen also judged nurses unable to respond to patients' needs in a timely way, and this was one of the prompts for her actions.

In a few instances participants in this study described working directly with health professionals to provide specific kinds of routine care. Ruth, for example, would often assist the nurses to turn her friend Kay in bed. Sometimes she moved to help simply because she was there, and not busy; in this way, her assistance was, as she says, 'automatic.' Yet it was also clear to Ruth that prompt nursing care for her friend sometimes relied on her own willingness and capacity to help:

> I'd say, 'it's time for her to be turned, she needs to be turned.' And they said, 'well, we're just in the middle of something, unless you want to help me, it's going to be like 20 minutes,' or whatever and I said, 'OK, I'll help you.'

Here, the allocation of caring work is made explicit, with Ruth agreeing to stand in for a busy health professional.

Like Ellen and Ruth, other carers in this study sometimes responded to conditions of health professionals' work by providing care themselves or working with professional staff. Also very significant were instances of family members and friends' working to secure care from health professionals. Strategies used to do this included trading services, becoming known, and progress chasing.

In several instances participants in the study spoke of 'helping' health professionals. As mentioned, assisting a nurse or physician was one of the ways that informal carers ensured that the ill person's care needs were met in a timely way. Other valued outcomes were apparent. Diane, for instance, perceived that the assistance she offered nurses was something they appreciated, and thus as a kind of trade for their professional services:

> The nurse would come in and say, 'oh, good, you're here.' I think they were more prepared to give her some extra time, maybe in the middle of the night if nobody was there, because they knew that during the day I'd be there. (Diane)

Dan also described caring for his wife throughout the night at the hospital. 'It helped them – understaffed and overworked and everything else,' he said. He then went on to link the nurses' appreciation for his help to subsequent interactions with them. Trying to sort through documentation about his wife's medication after she was transferred between hospitals, he phoned one of the nurses whom he had 'helped.' He described his pleasure that she remembered his first name, and commented on how she dealt with his request: 'it was almost like having personal service or whatever, but she immediately went and got what we needed.' Informal carers' 'services' to nurses, especially important in relation to their difficult working conditions, were seen to facilitate future goodwill and responsiveness to future care needs.

Almost without exception, participants in this study commented on the value of being or becoming known as an individual to health professionals. Being known was linked in respondents' experiences to swift responses by health professionals to care concerns. Frank's description of an oncologist saying that he would 'like to start chemo immediately' – even prior to certain test results, Frank notes – was followed by a passage about the esteem in which the medical team had held his wife. Martin, recalling a time when an outbreak of a hospital virus halted patient transfers between sections of the hospital, notes that he made a deliberate point then of telling nurses on the palliative care ward that a family wedding was on the horizon. Martin's wife was promptly transferred, and, as Martin said, 'had we been silent, had it been just another patient going to transfer, we wouldn't have gotten there then.' Martin saw his action of alerting the nursing staff to the upcoming wedding as elevating his wife from being 'just another' patient, just 'number 62 being transferred,' as he said later.

Several respondents set the value of being known against representations of hospitals and healthcare systems as factories, full of routine, and impersonal. Ruth, for instance, commented on the kinds of perfunctory caring that she witnessed, occasioned, as she suggests, by nurses' working conditions:

> Sometimes they just, and I realise they're busy and everything, but they almost do it by rote, or they do it, it doesn't / There's just not that emotional investment, it's just some body to turn. That's what it is.

Both Carol and Ruth described instances where ill people became 'just bodies.' 'Just a body' receives care devoid of empathy; 'just a number' waits for care. Being known, it seems, acts against prevailing conditions in health systems to secure care that is both emotionally engaged, and swift.

'Progress chasing' was a term used by a study participant, Martin, to describe his relationship to the health professionals involved in his wife's care. As he put it, 'progress chasing is, you know, we got this to do next, OK, well, is it happening?' Progress chasing includes the actions of monitoring the ill person's condition, tracking care schedules, and tracking down health professionals to address discomfort or to provide routine care. Sometimes family members and friends described their 'progress chasing' in quite offhand ways. In other instances participants outlined very active and conscious attempts to understand symptoms and care routines. The attention an informal carer devoted to monitoring the ill person and her care was sometimes explicitly connected to an awareness of nurses' working conditions:

> I have notes of every day ... everything. How many pills she's taken, when did she have a bowel movement, colour of her skin, temperature, everything. Because they [nurses] can't. They got 110 patients.

Progress chasing was a responsibility that every person who took part in this study in different ways took on. Yet it was clear in respondents' accounts that the activities associated with progress chasing could easily lead to them being perceived as demanding or needlessly anxious about the patient. 'The only thing I didn't want to do is bug them if they were busy,' said Ruth, reflecting the sentiments of several respondents. Yet informal carers, at the ill person's bedside, are acutely aware of care needs and the cost to the ill person of those needs going unmet. Ruth's friend, after a surgery, needed help getting to the commode:

> And so you're trying to help her out of bed and all that other stuff, and that's when you're supposed to get a nurse. And they would get a little exasperated at that because she was constantly thinking that she had to get up. But she also didn't want to pee the bed. You know, it was very ... that dignity being robbed from her, that independence. [pause] That was – oh man that was trying.

In comments like these, respondents captured one of the central contradictions of informal carers' roles. Informal carers feel compelled to 'chase' health professionals, because care needs would go unmet if they did not; and informal carers are at pains not to bother health professionals, because care might be withheld or compromised if nurses or physicians become irritated. When health professionals are 'run off their feet,' both the requirement and the risks of progress chasing are heightened. The possibility that care needs will go unmet is higher; so, too, is the possibility that health professionals will perceive informal carers' efforts to secure their attention and labour as demands.

Perceptions of Health Professionals' Working Conditions:
Effects on Informal Carers' Reports of Difficult Experiences

In speaking about the period in his life when he was caregiving, Martin described taking his wife to the emergency ward when she could not stop vomiting, and he feared she was becoming dehydrated. A few days prior she had had surgery on her back and then radiation. In the emergency ward, she spent over thirty hours on a gurney in the hallway:

> She was in so much pain … [long pause] You can't have anybody on a gurney with a back surgery issue for thirty-one hours and expect them to live … It was hard, it was a very, very difficult time. That was horrendous. That was just brutal.

In the wake of this experience, Martin's gesture towards the emergency room staff is, on the surface of it, barely fathomable: 'I wrote them a letter that was, I'm sure they still have it on the wall, I mean I tried to write them the most incredible letter to say, thank you.' His explanation for the letter: 'Because they did everything they possibly could.'

In this account an experience that could easily form the basis for an expression of considerable dissatisfaction is situated in talk in relation to health professionals' working conditions. In this process, something that might reasonably be expected from nurses – the timely securing of a bed for an acutely ill patient – is located beyond the bounds of human effort and will. It may well have been, of course, that not a single bed was available in the entire hospital. The point here is that it is quite possible to talk about this fact differently. Martin might have railed about his wife's (and his) suffering and blamed health professionals. Quite the opposite happens: in a situation Martin assesses as 'unbelievable,' the nurses also are described as 'unbelievable'; their actions exalted in the face of conditions in the health system deemed beyond their control.

Another participant in this study spoke about travelling with her partner to the cancer centre for a regularly scheduled meeting with the oncologist. When they arrived, the nurse told them the oncologist was not available and that another oncologist would see them:

> I was really annoyed about that and I said, 'you could at least call us and tell us that he is not here and let us make the decision whether we need to come and see another doctor.' And a lot of times it's not easy for the patient to come … And to come and not have your doctor there is just not acceptable to me in my mind. And I think that the least that they could do is give you a phone call and say, 'Dr. so-and-so isn't here, the other doctor is here,' you know.
>
> The other side of that in all fairness to the people at [hospital], at the cancer clinic is, it's packed. The cancer clinic is packed, and it's just … in the 6 years that I've been going to that cancer clinic it's gotten more and more and more. It's unbelievable to me. And so I guess really it's not feasible for them to call everybody on the day and say, 'well, your doctor's not here' which I mean, they'd probably be there all day, but I wish that there was something that they could do. (Ellen)

In the excerpts reproduced here, we can follow the course of Ellen's complaint. Early in the account the patient and carer occupy positions of entitlement in relation to health professionals: if the oncologist was not there, at least the nurse could call and let them know. Information about the unavailability of their regular physician is their right, and it is a health professional's minimal duty to ensure that right; the authority to decide whether they will see another oncologist is theirs as well. And yet, as Ellen says, the cancer clinic is packed. Set in relation to health system constraints, earlier assertions of entitlement are eroded. Initially claiming her right to a particular action on the part of health professionals, by the end of this passage the respondent is wishing for an undefined 'something' from them. The energy of her account dissipates and her complaint is disarmed.

The analysis outlined here is framed by the multiple meanings of 'disarm.' In the course of study respondents' narratives, critical commentary about healthcare and health professionals was often eased or pacified – disarmed – when health professionals' working conditions were taken into account. One of the narrower meanings of 'disarm' is also relevant here: to 'disarm' is to deactivate an alarm system.

Departures from Grounded Theory

Proponents of grounded theory locate its strength in conceptual density (Strauss & Corbin, 1994). Categories should be specified in terms of both properties and dimensions; a grounded theory monograph 'should be judged in terms of the range of its variations, and the specificity with which they are spelled out in relation to the data that are their source' (Strauss & Corbin, 1990 p. 255). In diagramming a conditional matrix to aid in the specification of conditions and consequences of a phenomenon, Strauss and Corbin note that conditions at all levels – from conditions in the international and cultural spheres, to individual action processes – have relevance. They contend that the researcher 'needs to fill in the specific conditional features for each level that pertains to the chosen area of investigation' (Strauss & Corbin, 1990, p. 162) 'regardless of which particular level it is' (Strauss & Corbin, 1994, p. 275).

It is in relation to the issue of 'levels' that I departed from grounded theory. In offering explanations for what happened with participants in my study, I did not seek to elucidate an exhaustive range of variations at the individual or interactional level. If I had, many factors – the length of time the ill person was in home and in hospital, the nature and extent of their symptoms and restrictions, the length of time between their death and the time of the interview, among others – would have earned a place in the analysis. My research aim was less to create a conceptually dense rendering at any particular level than to link aspects of the outermost circle of Strauss and Corbin's conditional matrix – culture and government – with individual actions, experiences, and narratives.

Over the course of my study, health professionals' (over)work emerged as a key link between that 'outermost circle' – health system restructuring – and the actions, experiences, and narratives of informal carers. Health policy and politics become meaningful in the lives of informal carers through their awareness of health professional strain and overwork (Sinding, 2005). This awareness and its consequences have implications for equity and quality in care. In this study, caregivers' actions appeared linked to health professionals' responsiveness to the ill person; such responsiveness may thus be unequally distributed, accruing more readily to people with strong and well-resourced kin and friendship networks (Sinding, 2004). As well, it was clear that when family members and friends of ill people see health professionals doing the best they can in difficult circumstances, they sometimes swallow their concerns about care. As complaints are 'disarmed,' inadequacies of care and attention go unrecorded and the call to collective action that might be provided by carers' experiences remains unformed (Sinding, 2003).

Acknowledgments

My appreciation is extended to each person who took part in this study. I am grateful for comments from Jane Aronson, Heather Maclean, and Ross Gray on an earlier version of this paper. The research presented here was supported by the Canadian Breast Cancer Foundation, Ontario Chapter.

REFERENCES

Charmaz, K. (1983). The grounded theory method: An explication and interpretation. In R. Emerson (Ed.), *Contemporary Field Research: Procedures, canons and evaluative criteria*. Boston: Little, Brown.

Charmaz, K. (1990). 'Discovering' chronic illness: Using grounded theory. *Social Science and Medicine, 30*(11), 1161–72.

Coburn, D. (1999). Phases of capitalism, welfare states, medical dominance and health care in Ontario. *International Journal of Health Services, 29*(4), 833–51.

Coffey, A., & Atkinson, P. (1996). Meanings and Metaphors. In *Making sense of qualitative data* (pp. 83–107). Thousand Oaks: Sage Publications.

Fakhoury, W., McCarthy, M., & Addington-Hall, J. (1996a). Determinants of informal caregivers' satisfaction with services for dying cancer patients. *Social Science and Medicine, 42*(5), 721–31.

Fakhoury, W., McCarthy, M., & Addington-Hall, J. (1996b). Which informal carers are most satisfied with services for dying cancer patients. *European Journal of Public Health, 6*(3), 181–7.

Glaser, B. (2004). Remodeling grounded theory. *Forum: Qualitative Social Research, 5*(2).

Heyland, D., Lavery, J., Tranmer, J., Shortt, S., & Taylor, S. (2000). Dying in Canada: Is it an institutionalized, technologically supported experience? *Journal of Palliative Care, 16* (October), S10–16.

Jarrett, N., Payne, S., & Wiles, R. (1999). Terminally ill patients' and lay-carers' perceptions and experiences of community-based services. *Journal of Advanced Nursing, 29*(2), 476–83.

Kristjanson, L. (1986). Indicators of quality of palliative care from a family perspective. *Journal of Palliative Care, 1*(2), 8–17.

Kristjanson, L. (1989). Quality of terminal care: Salient indicators identified by families. *Journal of Palliative Care, 5*(1), 21–8.

Kristjanson, L., Leis, A., Koop, P., Carriere, B., & Mueller, B. (1997). Family members' care expectations, care perceptions, and satisfaction with advanced cancer care: Results of a multi-site pilot study. *Journal of Palliative Care, 13*(4), 5–13.

Kristjanson, L., Sloan, J., Dudgeon, D., & Adaskin, E. (1996). Family members satisfaction with palliative care as a predictor of family functioning and family member's health: A feasibility study. *Journal of Palliative Care, 12*(4), 1–10.

Lofland, J., & Lofland, L. (1995). *Analyzing social settings.* Belmont, CA: Wadsworth.

Orono, C. (1990). Temporality and identity loss due to Alzheimer's disease. *Social Science and Medicine, 30*(11), 1247–56.

Payne, S., Smith, P., & Dean, S. (1999). Identifying the concerns of informal carers in palliative care. *Palliative Medicine, 13*, 37–44.

Rhodes, P., & Shaw, S. (1999). Informal care and terminal illness. *Health and Social Care in the Community, 7*(1), 39–50.

Seale, C. (1992). Community nurses and care of the dying. *Social Science and Medicine, 34*(4), 375–82.

Sinding, C. (2003). Disarmed complaints: Unpacking satisfaction with end-of-life care. *Social Science and Medicine, 57*(8), 1375–85.

Sinding, C. (2004). Informal care – two tiered care? The work of family members and friends in hospitals and cancer centres. *Journal of Sociology and Social Welfare, 31*(3), 69–86.

Sinding, C. (2005). Perceptions of oncology professionals' work: Implications for informal carers, implications for health systems. In D. Pawluch, W. Shaffir, & C. Miall (Eds.), *Doing Ethnography: Studying Everyday Life.* Toronto: Canadian Scholars' Press.

Skorupka, P., & Bohnet, N. (1982). Primary caregivers' perceptions of nursing behaviors that best meet their needs in a home care hospice setting. *Cancer Nursing, 5*, 371–4.

Strauss, A., & Corbin, J. (1990). *Basics of qualitative research: Grounded theory procedures and techniques.* Newbury Park, CA: Sage.

Strauss, A., & Corbin, J. (1994). Grounded theory methodology: An overview. In Y. Lincoln (Ed.), *Handbook of qualitative research* (pp. 273–85). Thousand Oaks, CA: Sage.

PART THREE

The Politics of Representation

6 The Stories We Tell: Processes and Politics of Representation

CHRIS SINDING, LISA BARNOFF, PAMELA GRASSAU, FRAN ODETTE, AND PATTI MCGILLICUDDY

The Lesbians and Breast Cancer Project was designed to generate understanding about lesbians' experiences of cancer and cancer care, and to foster positive change for lesbians with cancer in lesbian communities and in health and social services. We took a participatory action research (PAR) approach, in which researchers are positioned not as 'separate, neutral academics theorizing about others, but co-researchers or collaborators with people working towards social equity' (Gatenby & Humphries, 2000, p. 90). The Lesbians and Breast Cancer Project team was made up of lesbians living with cancer and lesbians affected by cancer; representatives from agencies in the cancer, lesbian, and women's health communities; and researchers. Twenty-six lesbians who had experienced a cancer diagnosis participated in the research, offering stories and insights about healthcare and social support, and about how their identities, bodies, sexualities, and relationships shifted and changed. *Coming Out about Lesbians and Cancer* is the report from the project. The full one-hundred-plus page report and a summary report are available as html files and for download in PDF at www.lesbiansandcancer.com. See also Barnoff, Sinding, & Grassau, 2006; Lesbians and Breast Cancer Project Team, 2004b; Sinding, Barnoff, & Grassau, 2004.

This chapter focuses on representation in two senses of the word – as it is used for those who participate in research and as it is used in the context of what researchers say about those participants.

The first sense of 'representation' has to do with those who participate in research. Marginalized groups have complex and sometimes brutal histories with researchers, sometimes exploited and experimented on,

Table 7

LESBIANS AND BREAST CANCER: A PARTICIPATORY RESEARCH PROJECT

Why was the research completed?
The study was designed to increase understanding of Canadian lesbians' experiences with cancer and cancer care, and to define directions for change such that lesbians with cancer might be better supported by service providers and lesbian communities.

What methods were used?
We took a participatory action research (PAR) approach. The project team was made up of lesbians living with cancer and lesbians affected by cancer; representatives from agencies in the cancer, queer, and women's health communities; and researchers. Twenty-six lesbians who had experienced a cancer diagnosis were interviewed, and offered stories and insights about healthcare and social support, and about how their identities, bodies, sexualities, and relationships changed with cancer.

The research and initial presentation of findings, in the form of the *Lesbians and Cancer Dialogues* was funded by the Canadian Breast Cancer Foundation – Ontario Chapter.

What were the key findings?
Participants told us that lesbian identity and realities are rarely addressed in cancer care. While most said they had not experienced homophobia, a few participants were targeted or denied standard care. A legacy of homophobia means that lesbians often work hard to secure good care, and can wind up grateful for the kinds of care that heterosexual women take for granted.

The study showed that the lesbian community unfolds in the lives of lesbians with cancer in complex ways. While most participants experienced robust community support, some reported isolation and disconnection linked to fear of cancer, homophobia in the broader community, and patterns of exclusion within lesbian communities. Many wanted a chance to connect with other lesbians with cancer. The project report, *Coming Out about Lesbians and Cancer*, is available at www.lesbiansandcancer.com.

What are some implications or results of the research?
To share the findings we created a staged reading of quotes from participants organized by theme: *The Lesbians and Cancer Dialogues.*

We have travelled with *The Dialogues* to cancer centres and communities in Ontario in partnership with the Canadian Cancer Society, Ontario Division.

  Many community initiatives were sparked or supported by this research, including:

- a support group for lesbians with cancer and one for lesbians and their partners
- a community program to promote access to breast health and breast cancer services for lesbians and bisexual women
- a website: lesbiansandcancer.com
- a video: *Coming Out Again: Lesbians Speaking about Cancer* (see the website, lesbiansandcancer.com)

commonly misinformed about the study purposes and risks, usually receiving scant direct benefit, and almost never involved in decisions about the research itself. Even when researchers clearly intend research to benefit communities, injustices and inequities persist. In research focused on lesbians and gay men, participants are often those most able to make their voices heard in all spheres of community life; the majority of studies rely on samples 'largely composed of white, middle-class, educated people with average or above average incomes living in urban areas, frequenting gay bars and identifying themselves as gay or lesbian' (Ryan, Brotman, & Rowe, 2000).

  The other meaning of 'representation' is 'portrayal.' In writing and speaking about research participants, researchers make countless choices. For the most part, we decide what is important about their stories and we say what their stories 'really mean.' Again, marginalized groups have often not fared well.[1] The extent to which research participants recognize their lives in researchers' words is questionable (Shope, 2006).

  These two aspects of representation preoccupied us as we engaged in a study about the experiences of lesbians diagnosed with breast or gynecological cancer. 'We' – the authors of this chapter – were part of the project team that guided and conducted the study.

Emphasizing Lesbian, Emphasizing Diversity among Lesbians ...

The project team suspected from the outset that things were less than ideal for lesbians with cancer in Ontario. Cancer care services were not exactly falling over themselves to increase their accessibility to lesbians. We thought we could use some research that identified lesbians as a community warranting focused attention from cancer care and support providers. Our research aim, then, was to explore and articulate the particular experiences lesbians have with cancer and cancer care.

The trick, of course, is that there is no such thing as 'the particular experiences lesbians have' with cancer and cancer care. Identities interconnected with lesbian, and structures of oppression intersecting with heterosexism, affect how lesbians respond to cancer and what happens to them. The kind and stage of cancer matters. As well, research participants' notions of what it means to be a lesbian varied, as did the significance they assigned to lesbian identity in their stories. Certainly we wanted to avoid essentializing lesbians – to avoid suggesting that 'all lesbians with cancer are, a, b, or c ...'

So we set ourselves this dual task: to make statements about the experiences of lesbians with cancer (particularly to reveal the operation of heterosexism and homophobia in cancer care) *and* to acknowledge the complexity of lesbians' cancer experiences. At moments along the way, however, we encountered situations and had insights that convinced us to emphasize one task over the other. This paper discusses those situations and insights; it is an effort to encourage, in ourselves and others, even greater consciousness about representational choices.

Leaning towards Diversity and Complexity

The project team knew that diversity mattered in many areas of life; we assumed it mattered in a cancer experience. In other words, we expected lesbians' cancer stories to differ in relation to social locations (race, class, age, place of residence, and so on). We wanted to engage the project work in a way that made it possible for these differences to come forward. In some important sense, we did not want our research to tell a coherent story. Discussing research with poor and working-class people, Michelle Fine, Lois Weis, Susan Weseen, and Loonmun Wong (2000, p. 111) note that:

> Although there is a class-based story to be told, a sense of class-based coherence prevails only if our methods fail to interrogate differences by race/ethnicity, gender, and sexuality.

In a parallel way, we believed that a coherent story about lesbians with cancer would prevail only if we failed to engage the multiplicity of lesbians' social locations. So we worked to recognize the complicated nature of the category 'lesbian':

- The project team was diverse in many ways. Membership included a lesbian living with a visible disability, a lesbian of colour, a lesbian with advanced breast cancer, a lesbian with gynecological cancer, the partner of a woman who had died of breast cancer, and lesbians of a range of ages. As well, the team was diverse in terms of the personal and professional experiences of its members.
- The project team developed a set of diversity goals, specifying in detail the diversity we sought in the sample (by race, income, education, age, ability, geographic location, identity, family status, time since diagnosis, cancer site, and cancer status). We developed a system to keep track of our progress towards these goals as we accrued participants and targeted our outreach specifically in areas where gaps were emerging.
- In our recruitment material, we deliberately attempted to reach out to women who did not identify with the term 'lesbian.' We were especially concerned that older women, who are more likely than young women to get cancer, might identify with other terms, like 'gay woman' for example. While we called ourselves 'the Lesbians and Breast Cancer project,' our recruitment flyers also said this: *'Labels – we can't live with them, can't live without them. By "lesbian" we mean women whose primary emotional and sexual relationships are with women.'*
- We know that certain communities of lesbians (for example, lesbians of colour, lesbians with disabilities, low-income lesbians) may distrust researchers in general, and be reluctant to be involved – in part this is because these groups are often not represented in research, or if they are, it is often in problematic ways. So our recruitment materials specifically stated our commitment to inclusion:

We intend to gather stories that represent the diversity that exists within lesbian communities. We plan to interview
- lesbians of colour as well as white lesbians
- older and younger lesbians
- lesbians with disabilities and able-bodied lesbians
- lesbians who live in different parts of Ontario in both big and small communities as well as rural areas

- lesbians who have primary breast/gynecological cancer as well as those
  with recurrence and advanced cancer.
  All lesbians are welcome to participate. *We especially encourage lesbians from
  equity seeking groups to participate.*

- Members of the project team took on focused recruitment with
  communities of which they were members – not because the rest of
  us expected them to 'represent' the entire community, but because
  we believed that lesbians of colour with cancer and lesbians with
  disabilities with cancer might be more likely to find the project credible because a lesbian of colour and a lesbian with a disability were
  active on the decision-making team.
- We developed community-specific recruitment materials. One flyer,
  for instance, read like this:

  Lesbians with disabilities, we want to talk with you!
  … It is important that we learn about how disability and lesbian identity
  come together when women with disabilities have breast cancer and that
  we look at the impact of ableism for lesbians with disabilities who have
  breast cancer.
       If you are a lesbian living with a disability and you have experienced a
  breast cancer diagnosis, we invite you to discuss the issues with us …
       Please contact us about how we can make this interview accessible for
  you.

- We undertook huge email and snail-mail campaigns with lesbian,
  women's health, social justice, and cancer agencies and used our
  personal networks to get the word out about the project. We also
  asked for advice about strengthening our recruitment approaches
  – for instance, we organized a meeting with lesbians connected to
  low-income and poor women to brainstorm ways to connect with
  lesbians with cancer living in poverty, and held teleconferences with
  health professionals and advocates across the province to understand how best to link with lesbians living in rural areas.
- We revised our research procedures where they seemed to present
  barriers – for instance, we initially asked potential participants to fill
  out and mail back a demographic form. Eventually we began doing
  the form over the phone, realizing that reading English or getting to
  a mailbox might be problematic.

So how did we do in our effort to engage the complexities of 'lesbian'? Certainly we did not access all the communities we had hoped to, to the extent we would have wished. Yet participants who identified with the non-dominant group were present in every category (see figure 6.1). Clearly barriers to participating in research are not overcome by representation (on the project team or in the promotional materials, for example) or by messages that researchers are committed to reflecting diverse stories. The issues are much larger and much more complex. For instance, homophobia in the disability community and ableism among lesbians undermine community building among lesbians living with disabilities. For some lesbians living with disabilities, then, lesbian identity may not be foregrounded. Lesbians who acquire a disability later in life, who were not previously confronted by ableist barriers to lesbian community, may have had greater opportunities to 'integrate' a lesbian identity. They may thus be more connected to lesbian community – and more likely to have learned about and participated in this study. Yet it is possible that these lesbians are less likely than lesbians born with a disability to articulate how ableism and living with disability can affect the experience of illness and care.

Some lesbians with disabilities who use attendant services, home care, or other care services may be especially cautious about coming out, and may thus be less likely to participate in a study like ours. This may be particularly true where attendant support is needed in relation to transportation to and from focus groups, or research events. Justice-oriented research designs obviously cannot entirely account for or respond to issues like these. Yet such research designs matter, and constitute steps towards more equitable participation in knowledge production.

Leaning towards 'The Lesbian Cancer Story'

In the exact time frame that we were directing energy towards recognizing diversity in this research, we experienced compelling shoves in another direction. During the recruitment phase, some key contacts – people we had hoped would assist us to connect with lesbians with cancer – strongly suggested that a study focused on lesbians with cancer was unnecessary and, in fact, unjustifiable. Sceptical questioning about how lesbians' cancer experiences could possibly be different from heterosexual women's came fast and furious, alongside firm as-

Figure 6.1 Participant demographics

Age	average age 50 (range = 36–72)
Diagnosis	breast cancer 22 gynecological cancer 3 (cervical 2, ovarian 1) One woman had both breast and gynecological cancer Cancer had come back after their initial treatment for 3 women, 2 of whom are living with metastatic (advanced) cancer
Time since diagnosis	3 years or more: 13; less than 3 years: 13
Place of birth	Canada: 20; United States: 2; England: 1; The Philippines: 1; Jamaica: 1; Hong Kong: 1
First language	English: 24; Cree: 1; Dutch: 1
Race/ethnicity (self-defined)[a]	Caucasian/White: 7; British: 6; Canadian: 2; Jewish: 2; Indigenous/Native 2; Metis-Ukrainian: 1; Euro Canadian: 1; Polish Canadian: 1; Italian: 1; Asian: 1
Total annual household income	100,000+ – 6 70–79,000 – 2 40–49,000 – 1 Less than 20,000 – 1[b] 90–99,000 – 1 60–69,000 – 3 30–39,000 – 4 80–89,000 – 1 50–59,000 – 4 20–29,000 – 2
Education	University degree: 19; College diploma: 6; Secondary school diploma: 1
Disability/health problems aside from cancer	One woman has a hearing disability; one has heart problems and arthritis and is a psychiatric survivor; one has experienced depression and has fibromyalgia; one has endometriosis
Urban/rural (at time of treatment)	Urban: 20; semi-urban: 2; rural: 4
Family status (at diagnosis)	Partnered: 17; Single: 9. Adult children: 5; young children: 1; trying to have children: 2
Identity	Lesbian: 22; Gay: 2; Dyke: 1; Bisexual: 1

[a] One woman said the question was impossible to answer as her ethnicity was "too mixed"; one did not respond.
[b] Actual income ~ $8000; one woman did not respond.

sertions that the experiences were not, and could not be, any different: 'cancer is cancer is cancer,' 'a breast is a breast is a breast,' 'cancer is the same for all women,' 'cancer is hard for everyone.' Lesbian identity and heterosexism were constructed as irrelevant. These responses were, of course, demoralizing. Underlying many such comments and questions is a conviction that lesbians do not deserve 'special' (that is, any) attention. Interestingly, lesbians are often constructed as 'other' until we demand more adequate services and resources – when we become, all of a sudden, 'just like heterosexual women.'

A key moment came at a meeting with another research team exploring social marginalization in relation to women's cancer experiences. We went to the meeting feeling very strongly that 'complicating the category "lesbian"' was the burning issue – indeed, we sought out this group of breast cancer survivors and advocates precisely because we hoped they would offer connections to women marginalized by structures of oppression beyond homophobia and heterosexism. The reactions of the other research team to our study were, however, similar to those described above.

As we debriefed that meeting, several things happened. We came to realize how common it is – especially when a health crisis looms – to deny that difference matters. In a sense, this censure of difference served to galvanize our own knowledge of how lesbian identity, and heterosexism and homophobia, do matter. We also came to the realization that 'complicating the category' could not always assume priority for us. Clearly, understanding that lesbian identity can be relevant to a woman's cancer experience is foundational to understanding the diversity of lesbians' cancer experiences.

When heterosexism is not acknowledged as a potential factor in lesbians' encounters with health professionals, for instance, it becomes pretty much impossible to talk about how heterosexism and classism might intersect in those encounters. What seemed most in need of articulation at that meeting (and in several other settings) was how lesbians' cancer experiences may differ from those of heterosexual women. It made sense to us, in that moment, to take a step back from our efforts to foreground complexity among lesbians, and to devote energy to the ways lesbian identity and experiences of heterosexism and homophobia affect women's experiences with cancer. We are aware that all of our research decisions are shaped by our own social locations. If the research team were all (or mostly) lesbians of colour, for example, different decisions may well have emerged.

The draw towards a clearly articulated 'lesbian cancer story' came not only from people outside the study; it also came from within. Once we had completed several interviews we created a draft community research report. Each section of the report began with broad brush-strokes, mappings, of the cancer stories lesbians told us and then narrowed to articulate the lesbian-specific features of the issue at hand. For example, the section on support began with a discussion about who offered support (partners and lovers, ex-partners and ex-lovers, friends – both gay and straight, children, parents) and described the kinds of support participants valued. Quotes highlighted instances of practical and emotional support, and made reference to the special kind of anticipatory guidance women who had themselves been diagnosed with cancer offered. Half way through the section, the focus narrowed to the particularly lesbian aspects of support; we noted, for instance, that some lesbians interviewed felt they were 'better off' than heterosexual women because their support was from women and specifically from other lesbians and was thus, they suggested, especially empathic and competently offered.

In keeping with our participatory framework we asked eight research participants to join the project team for two half-day meetings to review this draft report. At that meeting we received a strong message from them: 'we can read stuff relevant to *women* with cancer anywhere: you need to make the *lesbian* voice louder!'

This push to make lesbian 'louder' worried us for a few reasons. First, in their interviews research participants did not often make explicit connections between being a lesbian, and the kinds of experiences they had with cancer. We said this at the meeting, and the response was: 'of course they/we don't!' Sarah, a research participant, explained it this way:

[The interview] was the first time I got lesbian and breast cancer in the first sentence. So that was just an emotional interview. And as I sit back and look at this process and what the project means to lesbians, I'd like to be interviewed again, because I got the emotion out and I got my story out, and now what I need to talk about is being a *lesbian* with breast cancer. (Sarah)

Another research participant, Maureen, said this:

In my case I don't have other lesbians who are survivors around, or I don't know other lesbians who've had breast cancer. And so I haven't really had a chance to explore issues that could come up that I haven't thought of, or [say], 'oh, that's happened to me too' but I didn't realize it was because I was a lesbian. (Maureen)

This gave us pause ... because we had gone into the project knowing how very few spaces have been created for lesbians with cancer to speak together – indeed, both the interviews and our own experiences as researchers revealed how significantly lesbian identity is dismissed in cancer care and support services, and how often attention to lesbians' concerns is resisted and refused. We should have anticipated in a fuller way the situation Sarah describes, where the emotion of having that long-denied opportunity to talk naturally supersedes a focused consideration of 'the lesbian issues.' And, perhaps even more to the point, why we would expect a lesbian with cancer who has never met another lesbian with cancer to be able to articulate a common ground for lesbians' cancer experiences, we're not sure ...

And, we continued to worry. We worried that in focusing intently on 'what's lesbian' about lesbians' cancer experiences, research participants for whom 'lesbian' is less at the fore in terms of identity and social life would be less well represented in the report. We worried that by foregrounding heterosexism and homophobia in cancer care, we might imply that all lesbians experience heterosexism and homophobia similarly – that, for instance, lesbians of colour experience heterosexism in the same way white lesbians do. Yet in the context of the resistance we were witnessing ('cancer is cancer is cancer') and in response to clear direction from the eight research participants who participated in meetings to review the draft report, it made a great deal of sense to 'make the lesbian voice louder.'

From two quite different directions, then, we were pushed and drawn towards what Sherene Razack (1998) calls 'strategic essentialism.' Razack makes the point that every group is composed of members who are both dominant and subordinate. She argues that while it is theoretically (and at times practically) important to attend to multiple identities and multiple oppressions, there are times when highlighting this complexity might not be the most effective *political* strategy. She argues that it is sometimes more effective – when one is 'seeking to end specific hierarchies at specific sites' (Razak, p. 161) – to foreground one identity or form of oppression.

So, in our situation, for instance, we knew that lesbians living with disabilities face very fundamental barriers in cancer detection and care – as fundamental as inaccessible examination tables and mammography equipment. We knew from our study that middle-class lesbians were less likely than poor lesbians to speak about the costs – and thus the inaccessibility – of some cancer support services; poor lesbians also experienced class-based social exclusion in their interactions with physicians and other women with cancer. Similarly, we suspected that the intersection of racism with heterosexism would create distinct experiences for white lesbians with cancer and lesbians of colour with cancer. And yet we came to believe that focusing attention on differences in lesbians' social positions and experiences was at times not the smart or effective thing to do. In certain circumstances it made more sense to put our energies into articulating 'lesbians' cancer experiences' – to strategically essentialize 'lesbians' – in order to address the significant lack of understanding about how lesbians' experiences may differ from those of heterosexual women, and thus to offer a focused challenge to heterosexism and homophobia in cancer care.

Razack's (1998) analysis offered us a way of understanding our choices in the research process. It also reaffirmed the decidedly political nature of our study: it had social change objectives and required collective engagement. Participatory action research (PAR) clearly acknowledges that researchers cannot effectively describe injustice or champion change alone. As a collective of lesbians we were able to return to the interviews and create an analysis of how lesbian identity and homophobia mattered to cancer and cancer care much more effectively than any researcher could have done on her own.

Leaning Back, towards Diversity and Complexity

Razack's (1998) 'strategic essentialism' offered a critically important framework for our representational dilemmas. In part it pushed us to recognize the moments and situations when essentializing lesbians made good sense. Just as significantly, though, it challenged us to be strategic about *not* essentializing lesbians – to take full advantage of the moments where we could reasonably assume that audiences understood how lesbian identity and heterosexism/homophobia could matter to cancer experiences. In our own research reports, then, we made deliberate efforts to highlight diversity and complexity as clearly and as fully as the interviews we had done would allow.

Our central problem in attending to diversity in our research reports was that we had drawn a relatively privileged group of lesbians with cancer to the study. Where we did have narratives highlighting diversity among lesbians we focused on them carefully, working to draw attention to structures of oppression intersecting with heterosexism. In this effort we drew on the analysis emerging from the Ontario Breast Cancer Community Research Initiative's Intersecting Vulnerabilities research program, a program exploring how cancer care systems can create barriers to visibility and access for low-income, Aboriginal, and older women (Sinding, Gould et al., 2004). One of the participants in the Lesbians and Breast Cancer Project, Glenda, allowed us particular insight into these processes. Glenda told us about this encounter with a social worker:

> [The social worker] said to me, 'I can only work with you and your cancer, you've got too many things going on …' I was too poor, I was too busy figuring out what I was going to eat.

Glenda's experience, and her analysis of it, offered us a way to highlight processes of exclusion that echo across forms of marginalization. In the research report, we wrote this:

> services compartmentalize women's lives – as is so clear in Glenda's experience, where the social worker was only willing to talk with her about her cancer, even though her experience of cancer was intimately connected with her experience as a poor woman. For so many women, an experience with cancer cannot be separated out from oppressive realities, and complex identities. These realities and identities must be part of a service or program for it to be genuinely accessible for all women with cancer. (Lesbians and Breast Cancer Project Team, 2004a, p. 78)

We also drew from Glenda's comments and the story of another participant, Theresa, to offer a critique of how cancer support agencies construct their mandates. After having come out in a support group and experiencing negative reactions from other survivors, Theresa asked the group facilitator to talk with group members about different (that is, same-sex) relationships:

> [The facilitator said], 'well, it's really not my mandate … it's for the group to talk on its own and for me to give guidance, right?' And I go, 'so, what you're saying is, you're not willing to help me integrate into the group, right?' (Theresa)

In the research report we linked these two experiences – the hetero-sexist 'not our mandate' response Theresa heard with Glenda's classist 'not our mandate' encounter. We wrote this in the report:

> The notion that lesbians and poor women are 'not our mandate' clarifies the position of many cancer agencies: they do not deliberately or con-sciously exclude anyone, but lacking a critical perspective on their own services they wind up excluding lesbians and other marginalized women. … heterosexual, middle-class, white, able-boded women are at the centre of what they do; it is these women's realities that define the scope of many cancer care and support programs. (Lesbians and Breast Cancer Project Team, 2004a, p. 78)

In our critique of how agency mandates are defined, we are able to highlight some of the common workings of oppression. As well, in pointing to the embeddedness of cancer experience in all aspects of identity and social location, we are able to again lean towards revealing the complexity and diversity of lesbians' stories of cancer.

We also worked to highlight complexities in lesbians' experiences less clearly related to social location. Both to adhere to principles of qualitative analysis (Seale, 1999) and to minimize the risk of reinforcing dominant conceptions of marginalized groups (Shope, 2006), we delib-erately read for instances where participants' experiences or commen-tary departed from or challenged an emerging theme. So, for instance, in discussing findings about how lesbians' experiences of hair loss are shaped by lesbian 'culture' and community standards, we wrote this [the transition in the analysis is italicized]:

> Many women diagnosed with cancer cut their hair short before chemo-therapy. For some of the lesbians who participated in this research, having very short hair, a shaved head or being bald was linked with a positive lesbian identity:
>
>> I have a wonderful butch lesbian friend who taught me how to do my hair with one of those hair-clipper things. I had never done that before in my life. [laughter] And as a [professional], I always struggled with, 'OK, so, how dykey can my hair go and still pass, still be acceptable …' So it was the first time I could have a legitimate absolute dyke haircut. And so for me it was liberating … [and] sort of in tune with, we're queer, we're here, and we're not going away! (Marcia).
>
> Mary Lou spoke of a similar experience; after her hair grew back, she con-

tinued to shave her head. 'It's given me the freedom just to go – it's given me the excuse to be able to look, well, to look butch!' Paddy said, 'the cutting of my hair essentially was my way of saying to the world, 'I'm still a butch' in the face of the threat from cancer. In these women's stories, having very short hair was a way of affirming a lesbian or a butch identity and a way of maintaining or connecting to power.

Constance spoke about another connection between hair loss and being a lesbian with cancer:

> [In the queer community] they're like, 'yeah, you go girl ...' I still have one waiter at [restaurant] who always says, 'when are you going to shave your head again, I love that, you look so great.' I finally told him a couple of months ago why I didn't have hair then, he went, 'really, well you still look fabulous' and I thought, 'love you.' That was the kind of support we got, you know.

In queer community, Constance suggests, a bald woman is not necessarily seen as a woman with cancer. This meant that Constance was treated 'like a normal human being.' Queer culture lends hair loss a wider range of meanings for women than does the dominant culture, a feature of community that may be a source of strength for some lesbians with cancer.

Yet some participants in this research found nothing good or normal or powerful at all about hair loss. Rosalie, for instance, loved her long hair, and found it 'so hard to go bald.' For Teagan, losing hair during chemotherapy was part of 'not feeling human.' And Laura said this:

> You feel like in a way you've died and been reborn. Your hair goes right down below the skin line, it takes months for it to even come back, I'd never seen my bare head since I was a baby, and ... Oh, it was dreadful, I hid away from people. I hibernated, I was away from everybody ... If they would have said, 'what's the worst time of your life?' I naturally would say, 'when I was on chemo.'

While a lesbian identity might allow some women to buffer the difficult impact of hair loss, or even to find power in it, it was also clear from this study that hair loss can disrupt identity and be traumatic and disempowering for lesbians. (Lesbians and Breast Cancer Project Team, 2004a, p. 34)

The message here is that lesbians' cancer experiences are in some ways particular (as in, distinct from those of heterosexual women). As we note, in lesbian culture and community baldness has more positive meanings than it does in the dominant culture. Yet! – and it's an important yet – not all lesbians (even those with similar social locations) will experience these broad brushstroke characterizations as true or accurate. In a parallel way, the study report notes that lesbians commonly perceived themselves as 'better off' than heterosexual women in terms of social support, citing instances of immensely competent and loving responses to their illness from other lesbians. And yet! – most lesbians who took part in the research also experienced at least some instances of feeling and being isolated and disconnected from their partners, and from the broader lesbian community, a point we highlight carefully in the report.

The role of life-threatening disease in flattening, submerging, trans-forming, or highlighting identity, care, and coping is a thread that weaves throughout this project – as does the witnessing of the partici-pants' experiences of the recurrence of cancers and of death, and the angst of partners, children, and friends. Each woman who took part in this project brought a unique story – and that uniqueness is, we trust, visible in our work together.

Yet as researchers writing and speaking from this project (especially to health professional audiences) we often tell a 'lesbian cancer story' that depends on an over-coherent notion of 'lesbian,' rarely complicat-ed by intersecting identities – by which we mean, we mostly tell the story of lesbians with cancer who are relatively privileged. Our recruit-ment efforts drew a fairly homogeneous group; we feel certain that the narratives of lesbians with disabilities, lesbians of colour, older and rural lesbians diagnosed with cancer are more distinct than we were able to know from the stories presented in the report. We also chose in various ways to essentialize lesbians, and to assign lesbian identity more centrality in the cancer story than some participants likely would have done; with respect to the latter, the cancer itself, the challenge of mortality, assumed a particular centrality and preoccupation. Again, at this point in history and in the Ontario cancer care context, we can jus-tify our choices – and, we look forward to a time when they are utterly indefensible.

Acknowledgments

See page 229 for a listing of participants in Lesbians and Breast Cancer: A Participatory Research Project.

NOTE

1 The way this section is written implies that we (researchers) are never our-

selves 'marginalized groups' – which of course is not so, especially not in this project. And yet whomever else we may be, as researchers we have the authority to create representations of research participants; this is part of the complexity and challenge of participatory approaches.

REFERENCES

Barnoff, L., Sinding, C., & Grassau, P. (2006). Listening to the voices of lesbians diagnosed with cancer: Recommendations for change in cancer support services. *Journal of Gay and Lesbian Social Services, 18*(1), 17–35.

Fine, M., Weis, L., Weseen, S., & Wong, L. (2000). For whom? Qualitative research, representations, and social responsibilities. In N.K. Denzin & Y.S. Lincoln (Eds.), *Handbook of qualitative research* (pp. 107–31). Thousand Oaks, CA: Sage.

Gatenby, B., & Humphries, M. (2000). Feminist participatory action research: Methodological and ethical issues. *Women's Studies International Forum, 23*(1), 89–105.

Lesbians and Breast Cancer Project Team. (2004a). *Coming out about lesbians and cancer*. Toronto: Ontario Breast Cancer Community Research Initiative.

Lesbians and Breast Cancer Project Team. (2004b). Silent no more: Coming out about lesbians and cancer. *Canadian Women's Studies, 24*(1), 37–42.

Razack, S. (1998). To essentialize or not to essentialize: Is this the question? In *Looking white people in the eye* (pp. 157–70). University of Toronto Press.

Ryan, B., Brotman, S., & Rowe, B. (2000). *Access to care: Exploring the health and well-being of gay, lesbian, bisexual and Two-spirit people in Canada*. Montreal: McGill Centre for Applied Family Studies.

Seale, C. (1999). *The quality of qualitative research*. London: Sage.

Shope, J.H. (2006). 'You can't cross a river without getting wet': A feminist standpoint on the dilemmas of cross-cultural research. *Qualitative Inquiry, 12*(1), 163–84.

Sinding, C., Barnoff, L., & Grassau, P. (2004). Homophobia and heterosexism in cancer care: The experiences of lesbians. *Canadian Journal of Nursing Research, 36*(4), 171–88.

Sinding, C., Gould, J., Mitchell, T., Fitch, M., Gustafson, D., & McGillicuddy, P. (2004). *Intersecting vulnerabilities: Gender, poverty, age, Aboriginal status in women's lived experience of breast and gynecological cancers*. Paper presented at the 7th World Congress of Psycho-Oncology, Copenhagen, Denmark.

7 If Cancer Has No Colour, What Can I Say? Negotiating Racism and Analytic Authority

JENNIFER J. NELSON

> The author allows a limitation of the cancerous and dangerous proliferation of significations within a world where one is thrifty not only with one's resources and riches, but also with one's discourses and their significations. The author is the principle of thrift in the proliferation of meaning.
>
> *What is an author?* Michel Foucault (1984)

This chapter explores the analytic implications and responsibilities inherent in a researcher's authorship of other people's experiences. In particular, it examines what it means to interpret and retell others' experiences across profound social, personal, and political differences and limits. I tackle a series of questions through a research project example that sits at the crux of these differences and problems. I do not 'resolve' the questions and issues so much as I begin to unpack their complexities and propose ways to think of them as implicit and embedded elements in a research process.

The Researcher

Entering the field of psychosocial cancer care as a sociologist with a background in critical race studies, I was interested in illuminating systemic barriers to access and equity for marginalized women. I set out with the assumption that racism, as an institutionalized form in Western societies, shapes or permeates all aspects of social life, in overt and covert ways. My general research interest was to examine the forms and structure of racism in the cancer care realm at this point in time

– how racism organized people's interactions with the helping professions and support agencies, how racially marginalized women negotiated the services they needed, and whether or not they were able to get their needs met. I was interested in how the terrain of breast cancer has been established as (mainly) that of white, middle-class, middle-aged, heterosexual women with families. I wondered about the experience of obtaining emotional and practical support when one is excluded from this terrain, and how women interpret that experience. I was eager to learn what they thought was going on, what discourses they constructed and employed to make sense of their experiences.

Early on, I was introduced by a nurse colleague to a group of women of colour, all of whom were long-time immigrants to Canada, all but one from the Caribbean. They had contacted my colleague as they were interested in participating in and/or finding out more about research on race and ethnicity in breast cancer. A number of them had established their own cancer support network, called the Olive Branch of Hope, in order to address the support and information needs of women of colour, and to provide a space where their religious concerns could be acknowledged and shared. We agreed to embark on a qualitative interview-based study (see table 8, page 140) to investigate the issues women of colour felt were salient in their experiences with cancer (Nelson & Agyapong, 2004). An advisory committee was formed, which included my colleague, the founders of the support network, and a woman of colour who was a breast cancer educator, and who also took on the role of interviewer. Some support network members participated in the research and some assisted in recruiting other participants for the study.

Of necessity, as I investigated their views of cancer care, support services, race, and racism, I reflected on my role as researcher, particularly with regard to differences in subject position. I am a white Canadian-born academic. While I come from a rural, working-class background, through education and my professional position I would now be considered upper middle class. I was not experiencing financial difficulty (where some of the women were). I have also never been diagnosed with cancer. In short, I could not claim to understand their experiences. This may seem obvious, but it is important to make explicit, as this consideration shapes what is (and is not) possible to say about my research and my participants. In this light, before I broach the research itself, I want to introduce the theory/methodology that informs my analysis.

Table 8

WOMEN OF COLOUR LIVING WITH BREAST CANCER: BARRIERS AND BRIDGES TO SUPPORTIVE CARE

Why was the research completed?
The support needs of women of colour and immigrant women are often overlooked in the breast cancer community, and there is rarely attention to how racism influences women's ability to seek help.

What methods were used?
This study consisted of fifteen interviews with women of colour who were survivors of breast cancer. They belonged to a support organization called the Olive Branch of Hope. This group became the hub around which other participants were recruited.

We formed an advisory committee, with two founders of the support organization, a nurse manager, a breast health educator (who also conducted the interviews), and the principal investigator. We asked participants to describe whether and how existing support services had addressed their needs, any barriers they had faced, and what resources they felt were missing.

What were the key findings?
Many participants had received inadequate information and support upon diagnosis; they did not see themselves reflected in the breast cancer movement, and often felt unwelcome in mainstream support groups. They noted that fear of encountering racism can impede one's ability to access services, and that mainstream services are generally centred around a 'model' – white, middle-class – patient.

Many women said they would prefer race- and culture-specific information and services; it is often a risk for a black woman to discuss personal problems in a white support atmosphere. Christian faith was also a central element, and women found it difficult to be open about their faith in white environments.

The research calls for a broader understanding of the historical and social contexts in which racial domination takes place.

What are some implications or results of the research?
Our advisory group has continued to work together: the lead investigator sits on the board of directors of the group. Research results have been presented at national and international conferences, to health

and research audiences, at events in the black community, and in community newspapers.

The project team created the first booklet in Canada about the experiences of women of colour with breast cancer, which has been widely distributed to hospitals and community groups.

This research project helped pave the way for two successful funding applications for the Olive Branch of Hope, and has led to a larger study, which examined the breast cancer information needs of various racialized groups.

The Terms

I work in a poststructuralist framework, and draw on the work of Michel Foucault, among others, to assert that knowledge cannot be unproblematically produced, assimilated, and employed in the service of social change without consideration of its relationship to power (see, for instance, Foucault, 1972, 1980; Kendall & Wickham, 1999). Given this, I will briefly define some terms that appear throughout this chapter.

A *discourse* is a group of statements that constitutes a set of understandings about a topic or phenomenon at a given historical moment. Discourses construct the topic itself and the meanings that surround it. Discourses also define and govern what can be said and imply or delineate what cannot be said about a phenomenon (Jørgenson & Phillips, 2002; van Dijk, 1993). For instance, what might be called the discourse of 'survivorship' in the cancer community produces a kind of meaning about living with cancer that includes statements about optimism, mental and physical strength, and the will to persevere against illness. The prominence of this discourse can make it difficult to speak about personal weaknesses, fears, or the desire to 'give up.'

In Foucauldian terms, the term 'survivorship' does not have an inherent meaning outside of discourse; therefore, we can say only that its particular common meaning, at a given time and in a given context, takes this form and has this effect. That some discourses come to be dominant, and are imbued with a sense of authority, is a function of *power*. Discourses can 'congeal' to create 'regimes of truth' – ways of viewing the world that become powerful and dominant, while their social and historical sites of production are obscured. They become 'common sense, taken-for-granted, axiomatic, traditional, normal' (Carter,

2000, p. 28). As a function of the authority of the survivorship discourse, one might come to accept the statement 'a positive attitude helps one to survive cancer' as *knowledge* or *truth*. This form of analysis is not concerned with proving or disproving the truth value of the statement, but rather with understanding how the statement is constructed through discourse: how people's talk about survivorship allows this meaning to emerge, and how the statement garners the power to dominate, to render other meanings *untrue* or *unspeakable* in a certain historical moment.

Power, it is important to note, is not something that is possessed or held in particular bodies or places, but it is employed by particular people in certain situations. This in turn may provoke reactions or resistance (what is sometimes called *counter*-discourse). For example, vocal members of the cancer survivor community deploy power in putting forth the understandings of survivorship that they most value – such power allows these meanings (articulated through discourses) to become established as knowledge. Power, which Foucault described as a 'netlike' mechanism enveloping social relations, circulates not only through individuals but through social institutions (Foucault, 1980). The news media and the education system are institutions through which a particular discourse might garner enough power to become dominant or commonly accepted.[1]

When I refer to racism as institutionalized, then, I am referencing sets of discourses about racial differences that have been imbued with power in Western societies, so that they have been accepted as truth. For example, a common discourse about 'violent young black men' has acquired enough authority to affect racial profiling and the over-policing of black communities. This doesn't mean that all people believe the discourse; there are critiques and resistant discourses in circulation. It does mean that the discourse is powerfully operative in society, and, importantly, that such forms of knowledge have consequences – they give rise to particular actions. To say that racism is institutionalized is to say, for instance, that the news media, the education system, the police, the law are largely complicit in, and function to construct and uphold, racist discourses.[2] (Again, this is not to preclude the pockets of resistance and critique that do exist). Because these discourses are powerful, they are able to influence and dictate actions; what we *know* informs what we *do*.

Discourse analysis, then, can allow us to examine how particular forms of knowledge come to be and to study their effects in concrete situations. Discourse analysis entails a close and critical reading of texts with attention to such things as word choices, the order of ideas, sentence structure, emphasis, and various other functions of meaning-making (Jørgenson & Phillips, 2002; van Dijk, 1993). A 'text' itself might be anything composed of language – a conversation, a book, a lecture, an interview. Foucauldian methodology both includes and moves beyond this kind of reading; it is ultimately concerned with the effect of discourse, with *practices* – with what is enacted or produced 'on the ground.'

Finally, I want to address the notion of subjectivity or subject position. Foucault rejected the idea of an essential self; he was concerned, instead, with 'how social beings come to be made into certain types of subjects … through various modes of seeing, knowing, and talking about the world' (Carter, 2000, p. 28). As social *subjects*, we act as 'characters' who conduct ourselves within the framework of discourses. The character, or subject, is produced through discourses and is historically and contextually specific. For example, Foucault's work examined stock identities such as 'the hysterical woman' of the nineteenth century or 'the madman in the asylum' (Hall, 1997, p. 45), much as I identified the 'violent young black male' as a figure – a fiction – that is constructed through current discourse. Bronwyn Davies (1997) has argued that to analyse such subjects makes apparent '[their] fictionality, whilst recognizing how powerful fictions are in constituting what we take to be real' (p. 272).

What this conceptual framework allows us to do is question the social circumstances, the discursive and material forces that shape both identities and practices in contextually specific ways. When I identify myself as a white academic, this is significant in the context of my research with women of colour as it speaks to my access to power and authority as I narrate their stories and make meaning of their words for dominant audiences – some of whom are in positions to treat research participants' illnesses or assist them with personal problems.

Discursive formations, then, also matter in larger social scenarios; they inform what is understood about subjects and groups within professional circles or disciplines. In the following section, I will briefly outline some historical issues underpinning research across racial and cultural boundaries. This is linked to key critiques of knowledge production in some research contexts, and outlines my concern with how 'culture' is often constructed and taken up in the service of treating and helping racialized minorities. These concerns elucidate the theoretical links described above: discursive regimes dictate what is seen as knowledge, power operates in and through discourse to construct truth and to inform what actions are taken. At this moment in time, discourses about different cultures play a key role in shaping medical and social scientific understandings of racialized groups. Such meaning-making does not take place in a historical vacuum, but at the convergence of specific research practices, epistemological frameworks, and socioeconomic realities.

The Context

Histories and Narration

From the outset, I was aware that the research would be encased in various interlocking histories. There is a history of exploitative medical research and practice upon communities of colour (Bhopal, 1998; Harrison, 2001; Gamble, 1997; Francis, 2001; Dennis, 2001; Watts, 2003; Eliason, 1999), and social science research is similarly implicated (Thapar-Björkert & Henry, 2004; Harrison, MacGibbon, & Morton, 2001; Lather, 1988; Fine, Weis, Weseen, & Wong, 2003). The group of women and I would inhabit a gendered, classed, and racialized historical landscape in which black women's exploited labour has made white women's privilege and socioeconomic success possible (Fellows & Razack, 1998; Glenn, 1992; McClintock, 1995; Collins, 1990). As such, exploring race issues from a feminist perspective means acknowledging that much white feminist 'progress' has taken place on the backs of women of colour.

At the individual level, this means, for instance, that my career advancement is bolstered by their willingness to offer their experiences as my data. It means that their immigration, which is a key component of their identities as outsiders to the cancer community, is also part of a political economy in which poor countries supply a steady stream of cheap labour for wealthy, Western nations. This economic landscape, realized largely through migrant labour in the domestic, sex trade, and other low-skill, feminized professions, positions women differentially, and unequally, in Western societies (Kofman, 2004; Parreñas, 2001).

These contexts, while broad and only briefly delineated here, locate the research encounter within a specific time and space; they serve as a canvas on which the research relationship is drawn. Within them, I consider when, where, and how to draw on what is a relatively privileged position in order to get a message across, as well as what is to be the content of that message. Although I consult the community group for feedback, I am usually the one narrating presentations that will take their perspectives to the largely white healthcare community. I'm usually able to state what I think is important, and frame it in the way I think it should be heard.[3]

Within these contexts too, I make decisions about the interview process. The choice to have a black woman do the interviews was not straightforward, and this method should not be seen to 'take care' of potential power differences between interviewer and participant. I did not hire the interviewer based on an essentialist belief that her racial background would override differences or preclude problems. On the other hand, I assumed from the outset that the women would not necessarily be comfortable talking to me. We discussed this at some length in the advisory group, acknowledging that the interviewer, regardless of who it is, will always influence responses, and that race is not the only confounder in this relationship, although it is always important.

Ultimately, following the sense of the group leaders, we went ahead with a scenario that we felt was most likely to facilitate comfort and ease of communication in this particular situation. It was also due in part to other similarities between the interviewer and participants: she was a breast health educator who was very familiar with the issues; she shared their Christian faith and might better understand their spiritual struggles; she had met some of the women previously, and her personality and skills were well-suited to the situation. At the same time, I attended group meetings to present the proposed study and met as many group members as possible; they were aware of my leadership on the project and I contacted them with project transcripts and results and to ask for any feedback they had.

Such decisions around identity and strategy are rarely clear-cut in a research situation fraught with power differentials, and I do not consider them 'resolved.' It *is*, often, a judgment call, but it is one for which we can consider a number of relevant and difficult factors, often in dialogue with participants or other researchers, and with regard for the specific group and context.

Research Reception and Culturalist Discourse

Researchers who attempt socially conscious, ethnographic work must also consider the context in which the research is to be received. In psychosocial oncology, issues of social inequality remain marginal at best. Where notions of 'difference' are employed, it is usually in the service of changes to professional practice to accommodate the needs of various groups through practices like 'cultural competence' and 'multicultural-ism' training (see for example, Fowers & Davidov, 2006; Xu, Shelton, Polifroni, & Anderson, 2006; Doutrich & Storey, 2006; Todd & Baldwin, 2006; Davis & Rankin, 2006; Raso, 2006; Bussema & Nemec, 2006, Berlin, Johansson, & Törnkvist, 2006). Given the increasing ethnic diversity in Canadian society, addressing the needs of different groups is important. However, as various scholars have pointed out, such training and the knowledge on which it relies are often problematic (Gunaratnam, 1997; Fassin, 2001; Burman, Smailes, & Chantler, 2004; Abrums & Leppa, 2001; Nairn et al., 2004; Jeffery & Nelson, 2008; Park, 2005).

Cultural knowledge is often taken at face value with little critical attention to researchers' or participants' roles in shaping not only the data but how it is heard, understood, conveyed, and transformed through our various theoretical and experiential lenses. Uninterrogated forms of *knowing* about cultural 'Others' are prevalent in psychosocial oncology research literature (Altman, 1996; Galambos, 2003; Leigh, 1998; Jackson et al., 2000) and in healthcare generally (Betancourt, Green, Carrillo, & Ananeh-Firempong, 2003; McKennis, 1999; Waxler, 1990; Shen, 2004; Mir & Tovey, 2002). Such work tends to focus on different help-seeking, screening, and other health behaviours, or on the level of knowledge of various groups, including the myths they believe about cancer as 'barriers' to care, which are attributed to the groups' cultures (Bourjolly, Barg, & Hirschman, 2003; Phillips, Cohen, & Tarzian, 2001; Kinney, Emery, Dudley, & Croyle, 2002; Guidry, Matthews-Juarez, & Copeland, 2003). This knowledge-generation often takes place in the absence of any analysis of power relations.

Further, in the last several decades, as many theorists have demonstrated, racism has come to be articulated through a language of cultural difference (Essed, 1991; Razack, 1995, 1998; Goldberg, 1993). While theories of biological inferiority are generally no longer acceptable, culture has come to provide the ground on which hierarchies can be discursively organized. *It's not them*, we now say, *it's their culture* (Razack, 1998, p. 10). Culturalism, articulated through culturalist discourse, is defined by physician and anthropologist Didier Fassin (2001) as 'the *intellectual figure* that reduces culture to mere essence and that makes culture an ultimate interpretation of human behaviour' (p. 302). For researchers concerned with systemic racism, the reification of this ideology raises serious alarm bells: Where is power, what conditions are making this particular understanding possible, and why are those conditions so rarely transparent? Further, what is this knowledge producing; what does it dictate that we *do*?

In response to the last question, Fassin (2001) provides an excellent analysis of how culturalist explanations can serve to overshadow more likely socio-political reasons for poor access to health services. For example, in one case study, he describes how health professionals and researchers attributed Indian Ecuadorian women's distrust of healthcare systems and failure to seek obstetric care to their 'backward' cultural beliefs. Fassin's analysis revealed the women's long, arduous journey to the hospital site, their meagre financial resources, their lack of childcare at home, and undignified treatment in the hospitals when they did attend by professionals who regarded them with racist aversion. Within a culturalist framework, professionals are not required to critically examine their own practices or the systemic inequities embedded in the institutions in which they work, and the racism and socioeconomic problems that more fully explain poor healthcare are not addressed.

Problematizing Knowledge

In healthcare settings, in which the medical model and notions of objectivity remain central, research that accounts for subjectivity is often devalued or measured against 'hard science' standards of validity (Mays & Pope, 1995), which are simply not applicable to human interaction in historically- and socially-specific settings. In order that their work be heard in such settings, it is often in the best interests of social scientists to follow positivist traditions, to gather and distribute what is seen as factual, replicable data. It can be a challenge to suggest that knowledge about social phenomena is not straightforward, not 'true,' that knowledge is constructed, and that it has consequences, as Fassin describes. However, it is important to signal these concerns by recognizing that, as researchers, we always make choices; we favour, highlight, elevate, overshadow, and reposition elements of others' voices and experiences – this is what representation means. We have particular lenses through which we view phenomena (I have pointed to some of mine) and in viewing it, we tacitly accept that we will exercise power in our choices to portray certain information in certain ways, whether we acknowledge it or not.

I am describing the differences, tensions, and contextual limitations within my project at some length, because they speak directly to the analytic problems in question, which should become apparent during my discussion of the data. These dilemmas illustrate that a researcher's analysis and the transmission of findings to the rest of the world involve processes that are profoundly power-laden.

The Data

For the purposes of this chapter, I consider the sections from interviews that are relevant to views about racism or race-related issues. During interviews, participants were asked about their experiences in support settings and when accessing health and supportive care services. In many cases, they raised specific points regarding how racism and cultural differences influenced their experiences. At times, they were asked about their views on these issues when they described a problem for which the explanation was uncertain, or were prompted to say more when they broached the topics of race and culture.

Participants often refer to support groups they had attended, including the Olive Branch of Hope's own group. Some women referred to information sessions or discussion groups at hospitals, their experiences of approaching organizations for help or information, or attending community-based programs. As can be seen from the data, various perspectives were expressed, sometimes within the same interview, all of which demanded careful consideration. In the next section, I will present relevant excerpts from the data. Following this, I will outline and expand on the particular tensions or problems these research results reveal.

The (Dis)Ordered Themes

Qualitative researchers commonly approach interview data by coding it, choosing themes, noticing trends or tendencies, noting the anomalies, the contrasts, or the unexpected. We also acknowledge that most bits of data fall under, call upon, or give rise to more than one theme or argument, and we struggle with how to make sense of it all. But what happens when the themes occurring within the same interview, even within the same passage of text, appear incompatible or contradictory? There is no set of instructions about how to deal with this problem. What I've done for the purpose of this chapter is laid out a slice of the data, with internal twists and turns intact, called the twists and turns by name, and *used* the examples to think about authorship, representation, and political choices. I have entitled each segment of data with several themes in order to show how the themes recur in different combinations and how they overlap. I have purposefully avoided separating out and grouping segments from each interview that illustrate a *singular* theme – because it would not have been true to the way the data emerged, and because the point is to show how the 'messiness' of the data shaped my analytic concerns.[4]

EXCLUSION, RACISM, OR NOT

An excerpt from Collette's interview reads as follows:

Q: And you didn't go back to [names area] to the support group?
A: No, I didn't go back. It's more or less … they were not friendly.
Q: … because they were not friendly?
A: No, I didn't go back. I was the only black person there really. They were more friends themselves – like, among themselves – there.
Q: So do you think it was *because* you were black?
A: Well, I guess so, I guess they can identify with themselves more than with me … That was how it is.

Like Collette, Rose spoke about feeling left out in an all-white support session:

A: I didn't go back. I mean, if you are attending a group and you don't feel as though you are a part of it – if you are not made to feel welcome – why would you want to go back?
Q: Was racism a factor?
A: It wasn't mentioned but that's always sort of very ambiguous. I mean nobody comes to openly saying 'we don't want you here,' it's just the way they treat you … Nobody is listening to anything you have to say and if there is nobody interested in what you're saying … the normal reaction is 'what I have to say is not important to them.'

Reasons for discomfort in other support settings were often less clear, or multiple. Winnie, a colon cancer patient, noted that she had stopped attending a white support group. She began to explain the problem as a racial one but also noted that the breast cancer focus didn't apply to her:

Q: How did you feel when you were there, did you feel comfortable?
A: No, it is a lot of whites.

Q: Is that why you did not feel comfortable?
A: ...what they were talking about did not really pertain to me ... [I
   realized] this is basically for breast cancer because they don't talk
   about other cancers ...
Q: Was their being white also a factor? ...
A: No, you know I have nothing against, against, whites ... I don't
   have that prejudice at all, but what I felt is like ... 'we wouldn't
   want to stray from breast cancer ...'

Winnie went on to note that support services specific to black women
were very necessary, due to both culturally different needs and the difficulties many have in being open about cancer in their communities.
She also noted that cancer organizations seem to be mostly white.

RISKS OF DISCLOSURE, HISTORICAL LEGACIES, 'RACE MATTERS,' AND
'RACE DOESN'T MATTER'
Rose identified a particular risk many people of colour feel around
talking about their problems with white people present. Support group
members often discuss issues around family dynamics, or how family
members are coping with their cancer. Since many white people hold
stereotypes of black families as dysfunctional, she felt that discussion
of any problems in black homes might be seen to reinforce these beliefs.
She also offered a historical explanation for why it might be difficult for
black women to find support:

> we were brought up to be private, black people are not generally people
> who go out and talk about their problem regardless of what kind of prob-
> lem it is. Colonialism helped with that! (laughs) ... So coming out and go-
> ing to a support group and talking about our problems in front of people
> of a different culture is not something that we are going to find too easy
> to do.

Paula also felt that people were often more comfortable talking about
personal issues among other members of their racial group. Like several other women, Paula stated that she had become interested in the
Olive Branch of Hope because it was specifically for women of colour.
However, she was somewhat self-critical on this issue, feeling that she
should be able to talk about her experiences regardless of the group's
make-up: 'I think I should be open at both places ... when we see one
another's condition – we are no better than one another.'

REPRESENTATION, RACISM, 'RACE DOESN'T MATTER,'
AND 'RACE MATTERS'

When asked about support services, several participants described a program that helps women cope with changes in their appearance during cancer treatment, through tips on skin care and make-up, for instance, as well as the use of wigs and head scarves. Those who had attended noted that many of the products they were offered were for white skin and hair. Candace criticized this aspect of the program, but she later noted that she did not feel racism was a factor in finding support: 'I don't think it is prejudice or because we are black or racism, I think it is awareness ...' When asked whether she thought it was important that a support group for black women be all-black, Candace expressed a fairly common belief among participants – that it was not necessary because 'anyone' can get sick and need help. However, she added that it was nice to know there was a black women's group available, as 'black folks will understand what we go through.'

Karen described attending the appearance-oriented service: 'I think it is important that they identify that not everybody is a certain colour ... like, I remember the foundation vividly – not having [my colour], not having the lip liner ... but I think the whole gesture was good.' Doris described having attended the same program, being the only black cancer patient at her session. She expressed concern about the lack of representation generally:

> even from what I have seen in magazines, yes – there may be a black woman, but the ratio of minorities to Caucasian women is very small ... I have not honestly seen or heard any black women as advocates for [the breast cancer organizations] ... Black women [are] different in the way they communicate their feelings; they do not normally walk into an environment and just express their feelings – they need a sense of identification. And first of all, it is obvious on a visual scale if a black woman walks into a room and they are the only black woman in the group; it is more than likely that they will be quiet ... if they saw other people of colour in that room there will be a sense of 'oh I am not the only one' or 'there are other people who look like me or feel like me.'

CULTURAL DIFFERENCE, 'RACE DOESN'T MATTER,' AND THE NEED
FOR SPECIFIC SERVICES

When probed further about black women's reluctance to seek support, Doris attributed it to cultural norms which encouraged black women to put their families' needs first, stating, 'it has been embedded in them that their needs are not important.' Frieda also stated that the black community had not progressed enough in speaking openly about cancer. She felt that black women need to be open about having cancer to raise awareness of the issue and their own needs.

When asked about the racial composition of support organizations, Frieda replied that she thought a racially diverse group was the best scenario because people learn best from exposure to a range of experiences. However, when asked at the end of the interview to sum up what she thought was important for black women coping with breast cancer, she emphasized that more support services for black women in particular would be useful, as well as support and information specifically tailored to black male partners and families of patients.

Emma did not speak of any experiences with other groups or services, but she expressed the idea that skin colour should not matter when people are coping with cancer.

Q: [I]f there were white ladies in the Olive Branch of Hope, do you think you would have felt this comfortable as compared with now that they are all black ladies?
A: I think I would have felt the same way because I think we are all one – not the same colour, but we are all human beings ... I think we are all one.

Marilyn noted that women of any race are welcome in the support group:

Q: Is it important that the group is all women of colour?
A: No... [We started a place] where we can be free culturally and spiritually but that does not exempt others and we don't impose our spirituality on anyone. The basis of anyone coming is for support.

She shared the common sentiment that black women had difficulty sharing personal experiences: 'We don't – and this is all cultural – we don't share things openly, you don't talk about your body parts openly, and so many find it necessary to keep these things quiet.'

Jean echoed the sentiment that people learn more from diverse groups and noted that she would prefer a 'mixed' support setting. She advised that women need to seek information regardless of the setting: 'it is true that you don't see a reflection of your community ... or other communities, but this should not hinder you from asking questions. [Women of colour] shouldn't be inhibited, they should be proactive.'

SOCIAL INEQUALITY, 'RACE DOESN'T MATTER,' AMBIGUITY, AND THE NEED FOR SPECIFIC SERVICES

At another point, Jean was asked whether she thought people's backgrounds could affect their ability to find support: 'Yes I think so because many women may be single mothers and may come from a different socioeconomic background and may not have ... things to do with people who are not of their colour, and may feel self-conscious.' She did not feel that support services for specific communities were necessary, however: 'because you know what I think? I think whether you are black, green or whatever, we are first of all human beings.'

When asked whether it had mattered that she was the only black person in a group she had attended, Karen replied that it wasn't important, because 'cancer doesn't have a colour attached to it.' The important thing, she felt, was finding support in a setting where one feels she belongs, regardless of the constitution of the group. As noted earlier, Karen had also expressed a concern with the lack of representation of black women. She stated:

> being a black person, you connect more with black people about certain things but ... a struggle is a struggle, a hurt is a hurt ... You know it is important to a lot of people that it'd be just for women of colour. I like the fact that, you know, I can go, you can go and you can be yourself, but if a white person wants to walk in I will be okay with that.

Beth joined the group several years after her diagnosis because the group had not existed at the time; she said that it would have been helpful to know about the group when diagnosed 'because it is for women of colour.' Beth later indicated that sharing would probably not be affected by race in a diverse group:

Q: But do you think that black women in the group will feel open enough to share – like they're sharing now with only black people in the group – if you had white ladies?

A: I think so because we are all, we all have the same sickness and we all need answers, we all need comfort, we all need support.

When queried about another group she had attended in the past, Beth seemed uncertain about her feelings around race:

A: It was mainly whites … all white, at the time, and I didn't feel I needed that …
Q: Was it *because* they were all whites?
A: Maybe – I think you feel comfortable or more comfortable with your own … you can relate more … although those that were there with me at the time were all whites and we were encouraging each other … but I chose not to [continue going].

HISTORICAL LEGACIES, SOCIAL INEQUALITY, RISKS OF DISCLOSURE, AND RACISM

Rose situated her views on the needs of cancer patients in historical context:

> The healthcare providers need to go out into the community and be able to communicate with the people. We live in an indigenous community and just to stay there and say 'you come to us' – black women aren't going to get up and go. I know it is easy for them to say the onus is on [the black women] … but we don't normally go because when we go to the health centres we are going to see white faces and it reminds us too much of colonialism so we don't want to be reminded so we don't go.

Grace, too, situated the culturally-specific issues facing women of colour within a broader socio-historical realm. She attempted to explain the protection of privacy in black communities:

> it is a cultural thing … and if we go back to slavery when our ancestors came to different countries as slaves, they had to be secretive … and so it comes down from that generation where we are always taught [not] to be too open …

Grace elaborated on racism in healthcare:

> One of the problems is that many people of colour find in hospitals and different places where they go to get treatment they are sort of treated different, they don't treat them the same as they treat the Caucasian, the other groups. Although we are uniquely different in our make-up as a person we

are the same and we like to be treated with respect, dignity as other nation-alities. And so they should have training, this should be part of the training for all health practitioners – from doctors right down to whoever clean the floor for them – should be educated in diversity training.

She continued to place the problem in a much larger social context:

Sure we are a guest in your country but many of us have been here for a long time – we have contributed to the country's economy in many ways … so therefore we will want our fair share of the pie in that we get respect, we get recognition and sure we would like monetary compensation too, some help when we cannot help ourselves after we put in our strength, our youth into the economy, then when we are sick … you know, those are the things that concern us and sometimes make you a bit angry, and you wonder, why can't we feel like we are a part of the society here? … [m]any of us, we brought our education, our skills here and even whatever we acquire we worked and paid for … contrary to the myth that we come here to get something … we are a very important part of the society but very few people know because it is not broadcast. You don't see the nice young men in university who have won scholarships and who are doing well, you don't see them on television, you see the ones in handcuffs and going to jail, that's all you see…

And So…

Of the fifteen women involved in the study, five participants explicitly named racism as an issue and two described a historical context for racism and current problems in their communities. Three of the fifteen expressed the view that women of colour were generally more comfort-able in support settings with other women of colour than with white women. Overlapping with the former category, eight more women seemed uncertain about whether they would prefer an all-black group for themselves. Five stated explicitly that race does not matter, express-ing, albeit in different ways, the notion that 'everyone is the same.' One participant did not raise issues or engage with questions about race or discrimination. Eight of the fifteen women attributed the lack of awareness and openness about cancer in the black community to black Caribbean culture. Five expressed some concerns related to race (repre-sentation, lack of diversity) while not naming racism, and only one said explicitly that there was not racism in her experience.

As the data make evident, most of the women's interviews fall under two or more of these broader themes. Moreover, some women expressed views that might be seen to fall on both ends of the spectrum; for example, those who presented a detailed anti-colonial analysis were not necessarily in favour of racially-exclusive/all-black support settings.

In emphasizing the range of opinions, I risk suggesting that diversity within the research sample is somehow surprising. And in describing some narratives that may seem to express contradiction, I risk suggesting that the women were mixed up or inarticulate. Neither is my intention. On the contrary, I did not expect to find a unified set of assumptions, experiences, or perspectives within the sample. At the same time, I was somewhat surprised to find such a range of views within individual interviews. I am interested in what this might reveal about analysing and representing participants' words.

The Problems

My work has been centrally concerned with the construction and productive influence of knowledge about racialized groups. Because I believe it politically necessary to anti-racist projects that experiences be explained in historical and social context, I was interested, for instance, in the views expressed by Rose and Grace, which incorporated a situated historical reading of current struggles. These women named what are often (problematically) called 'cultural barriers,' but they situated these barriers within a much broader set of socio-political circumstances: colonialism, slavery, immigration, and a history of racist representation in the North American media. Instead of reinforcing culturalist discourse, they called upon the ever-present dynamics of domination through which 'barriers' are created and sustained (Gunaratnam, 1997; Fassin, 2001).

Faced with largely white audiences of healthcare providers, researchers, students, and others, and armed with a series of statements from women of colour about 'the problems with black culture,' I had to think very carefully about what it was possible to say. I am acutely aware of the potential for fuelling the fire, making matters worse by providing 'evidence' that culture (theirs – not ours) is the problem. I felt it important that more contextual readings be centrally positioned in research accounts; still, I had to be attentive to the fact that not all participants expressed these views.

Statements to the effect of 'everyone is the same' also present certain risks: 'Whether you are black, green or whatever, we are first of all human beings' … 'We are all one' … 'A struggle is a struggle, a hurt is a hurt' … 'Cancer doesn't have a colour.'

Canada's national identity is composed of a discourse of tolerance and acceptance towards all cultures and races signified in a policy of 'official multiculturalism.' Such a policy operates overtly and covertly to suppress the acknowledgment of racism in Canada and to reinforce belief in the liberal rhetoric of equal opportunity for all. Similar to culturalist understandings, the discourse of multiculturalism can serve to conceptually flatten power hierarchies, insisting that we are all simply *different but equal.*

The participants, of course, want *all* women to receive help. So do most healthcare providers, researchers, and community groups. However, such statements can be read as indicators that all people should be treated *the same way* rather than treated *as equals* but with regard for their specific needs, and regard for the fact that they do not, in fact, have equal access to resources and opportunities. Cancer may not have a colour, but people do. My participants know this; however, white, 'multicultural' societies nurture 'colour-blind racism' which purports to deny the salience of difference in the name of equality, rather than acknowledge inequality as their bedrock (Yee & Dumbrill, 2003). This manifestation of liberalism also supports the notion that racism is episodic, rather than systemic. And so, in a forum in which 'diversity' as a concept remains new, and 'power' non-existent, I did not relish the idea of reassuring hospitals, professionals, community organizations, and researchers that really, things are all right as they are; there is no need to critically review our beliefs and practices, and differences do not, in the end, matter.

I resisted the idea that cancer transcends race and other differences – 'cancer has no colour' – that illness simply becomes a common terrain on which women can relate to one another as equals. To be clear, I am not suggesting that women cannot relate across differences at all (nor am I making any suggestion about the 'best' racial composition of support groups), but rather that these differences, and the broader issue of differential access to resources, cannot simply be subsumed or erased; otherwise, why wouldn't mainstream, generic support services work fine for everyone?

Besides my broader political concern around 'colour-blindness,' I felt that the women's narratives provided many other examples of how such transcendence was not possible. There were many ambiguities within interviews, where, for instance, examples of inequality were described even when discrimination was disavowed at another point When asked about the particular difficulties around cancer within black communities, Candace noted, 'I don't think it is prejudice or because we are black or racism.' Later, she was very critical of images in cancer information literature that portrayed only white patients and expressed the idea that black people would better understand her experiences. Also quite commonly, women expressed a view that everyone should be welcome and that differences shouldn't matter but later suggested otherwise. For instance, Frieda indicated that racially-specific services were unnecessary but then identified specific needs of black women that she felt were unaddressed. Beth noted that a diverse group would be more beneficial but later expressed discomfort about her own experience in a group of white women, which she had left.

Further, evident in this data is a fairly common view that the participants' support network should not 'discriminate' against anyone of a different ethnic background, including whites. Most of the women made it clear that anyone is welcome to join for support, and I read in this a sense that to exclude anyone would be considered wrong. Take, for instance, Winnie, who said, 'I have nothing against whites … I don't have that prejudice at all.' Other participants suggested that, regardless of their own views, many people do prefer that whites not be present. Comments like this taken out of context can be received within a conservative discourse of 'reverse racism' – the belief that anyone can be 'racist' against anyone. This flattens power hierarchies and suggests that all discrimination is the same, or 'equally wrong' – rather than framing blacks' negative feelings or desire to avoid whites in some instances as a rational response to the histories that Grace and Rose highlighted – of colonialism, racist representation, slavery, and socioeconomic oppression. Such responses are constituted within a set of power relations that, by definition, make them *not* the same as racism.

Another important issue differentiates the participants' discourse around inclusion: to say that white women are welcome or that it would be 'okay' for whites to attend a group does not necessarily alter the fact that the women of colour who form the group remain the *hosts*, nor that the group has been designed to centrally address their concerns. The group remains centred around the concerns of women of colour, no matter who attends. This is a political shift from dominant modes of cancer support in which white mainstream concerns are centred to the exclusion of others, or in which marginalized women's concerns are 'added on' in a token manner.[5]

The women were quite clear that they did not want to replicate exclusionary practices – the answer to discrimination is not more discrimination. At the same time, many of them noted that there were things they wouldn't be comfortable discussing with whites present. Some of them seemed uncertain as to the reasons they discontinued their attendance at mainstream services; some pointed to exclusion that seemed implicitly racist, but was not overt enough to name. It is possible that some were self-conscious about expressing negative feelings towards whites because of me. Even though the interviews were conducted by a black woman, they knew that I was the principal investigator and many of them had met me. They were generally eager to make me feel welcome at group events and some explicitly told me never to hesitate attending because I was white. It is also possible that some maintained a cautious attitude towards the study because it was conducted through a hospital where they received treatment. Although they had no direct contact with the institution as part of the study, consent forms appeared on hospital letterhead with research ethics board contact information.

Precise definitions of what constitutes discrimination or racism were not broached in the interviews. Some participants may not think of lack of representation or of programs with products only for whites as 'racist.' It can still, I would suggest, be argued that a problem is present in such examples, and that the problem lies on a continuum of exclusionary practices and events that are underpinned by systemic racial inequality. What appear to be innate cultural patterns develop in and through historical circumstances. Thus, the examples that account for colonial histories do not contradict the other women's comments about black cultures being 'at fault'; rather, they explain them in a particular way and place them in a larger context, which also leaves room for other views about representation and exclusion that might seem discordant.

The notion of a continuum helps in making sense of what seem to be contradictions or ambiguities in the interviews. It focuses attention on how racism operates in social life, through institutions, including hospitals and community organizations, in ways that are often covert. By considering further external factors – for instance, that the researcher's subject position and the presence of institutional authority in the research process may influence participant responses – I am expanding this continuum to make space for responses that would disavow racism, while still acknowledging that power relations are present. Expressions of uncertainty, discomfort, or more vague recollections of feeling 'out of place' signal the importance of a close discursive reading that considers what it may be difficult or impossible to say, as well as what is said. It is not necessary that explicit examples of discrimination be articulated in order to 'find' race and racism in the text. This points, again, to the potential risks of simply leaving the data to speak for itself, particularly when presenting it to dominant audiences. Such a face-value reading may miss nuanced or more subtly articulated problems that are, when placed in context, not as benign as they seem.

In analysing the data in a particular way and choosing to highlight and emphasize aspects of it, I am also choosing to position it politically for what I hope is a progressive educational end. An alternative would be, as I mentioned earlier, to highlight the responses that seem to implicate black culture in women's problems with services. This, too, is an exercise of analytic authority, with a potentially very different social/ political outcome. In highlighting particular views, I risk the accusation of 'cherry picking' – choosing to present only the data that supported the arguments I wanted to make. I challenged myself to look at, and write about, the range of viewpoints identified. I chose to acknowledge that my own political position is better reflected in some accounts than in others, and to say why I think those accounts provide a necessary context, especially given the audiences who will consume the data. In addition, I offered my own contextual analysis, pointing to some of the history that forecasts my engagement with this group of women, and drawing on scholarship that has documented this history. With some trepidation, I decided to point out the potential harm in simply letting the data speak for itself. This is not to say that this 'takes care' of potential misreadings; it *is* to say that the researcher always makes choices, so, at the very least, we can make those choices transparent.

By emphasizing the existence of a systemic underlying racism while some participants would disavow it, I might be accused of suggesting that the women have 'false consciousness.' This is a Marxist term, thought to have been articulated primarily by Friedrich Engels, that describes the absorption of dominant ideology by the working classes so that they're unable to recognize their own oppression (Westby, 1991). I am not suggesting that my participants are unaware of racism – and certainly not that I am better versed than they in its manifestations and effects. What I would suggest is that their responses, whether they deny or confirm racism (or are ambiguous and fluctuating, as so many were), actually attest to the difficulties of race, of pinning down its meanings and discerning its shape in social relations. They point to the continuum of experiences, articulations, confusions, harms, and resistances that histories of enslavement, racism, and displacement make possible.

Their responses amply illustrate a profound underlying problem: that women of colour can't choose *not* to think about race. They need to wonder why they don't feel safe; they need to assess their environments, adapt available resources, decide if and what to disclose to whom. They wonder if their sense of exclusion is fair or correct; they worry that they've got it wrong; they challenge themselves to 'come out' regardless of their audience and not to replicate exclusion and discrimination. They critique racism; they doubt racism; they are concerned about their own representation; they are concerned about its effects on other women; they assert culturally-specific needs; they question their cultures; they think critically about dominant culture; they want their needs and the needs of their families addressed; they want to recover. They also negotiate illness and racial meanings in a historical terrain marred by powerfully enduring stereotypes – of the domineering, castrating black woman, the welfare mother, the idealized, complacent 'mammy' who nurtures everyone else (Taylor, 1999; White, 1985; Glenn, 1992; Higginbotham, 1992), and the shiftless and violent black male (Gilroy, 1987).

Their struggles fall along a continuum of critique-acknowledgment-uncertainty-disavowal of racism. Together, they compose a social scaffold from which they describe and prioritize the nature and forms of their support needs differently and in different times and places. But all the dimensions of experience, replete with contradictions and overlaps, exist within a larger framework in which racialized bodies are read differently than dominant bodies, in which racial groups are ranked, and in which political struggles and history and violence shape what it means to be a woman of colour who is trying to survive.

The (sort of) Conclusions

To examine racism in cancer care experiences is not to assert that it overrides all other factors in people's lives or that it has the same impact on everyone. When understood as a systemic organizing principle of Western societies, racism is not simply attributed to individuals (although individual practices may very well be implicated) or located in isolated acts (although those acts do take place). Rather, a systemic approach makes clear that the same factors, questions, fears, and dilemmas that structure any experience or encounter will be present as a woman visits a hospital, makes decisions about surgery, goes to a support group, visits a health library, or reads breast cancer information.

Similarly, the same power relations will be at play as we do research, learn about our data, and present research results. We will face questions of context, subjectivity, voice, and the challenge of how to best frame issues for particular audiences depending on the outcomes we hope to achieve. As Fine, Weis, Weseen, & Wong conclude about their own research setting, 'We need to invent an intellectual stance in which structural oppression, passion, social movements, and evidence of strength, health, and "damage" can all be recognized and theorized without erasing essential features of the complex story of injustice that constitutes urban life in poverty' (2003, p. 125).

I began by noting that this discussion would not provide conclusive answers. In fact, I think it's important not to attempt a recipe for 'doing it right' precisely because each research project is context-specific. Methodologies are not intended to be static and generalizable; they are tools to be employed as needed and adapted to different phenomena. I don't feel I have done it 'right'; nor have I necessarily done it 'wrong.' In this discussion, I have employed some tools for thinking critically and contextually about data that span a number of important social differences. I have suggested considerations for how we think about knowledge – what constitutes knowledge, what dangers are inherent in propagating particular forms of knowledge about other people as we attempt to represent our data, and what it may be useful to think about as we go about doing this.

Further, as I've hoped to show, being reflexive means more than naming social locations and identities; it means asking critical questions about how we think, how we define knowledge, what it is possible to know, and what is important to know. It is about remaining aware of our reactions to, for and against, our data. There will always be old and new analytic tensions, questions, and continued differences to work out – or not work out. But at the very least, I have hoped to illuminate some ways of making these traps and troubles discernible, of accepting the difficulties as part of the research process, and of possibly doing it better in the future.

Acknowledgments

WOMEN OF COLOUR LIVING WITH BREAST CANCER STUDY
Principal Investigator: Jennifer Nelson

The Project Team: Florence Agyapong, Immigrant Women's Health Centre; Leila Springer & Winsome Johnson, The Olive Branch of Hope breast cancer support services; Sherrol Palmer-Wickham, Toronto Sunnybrook Regional Cancer Centre.

This project was funded by the Ontario Breast Cancer Community Research Initiative, which was funded by the Canadian Breast Cancer Foundation, Ontario Chapter. I am grateful to my co-editors and to Donna Jeffery for their comments on earlier versions of this chapter.

NOTES

1 For a Foucauldian reading of the construction of subjectivity in the education system, see Popkewitz, 1998.
2 For examples of studies focusing on law and historical racist discourse in the Canadian context, see the collection, Razack, 2002.
3 In spite of attempts to maintain a participatory framework in the research, it is sometimes the case that women lack the time, resources, or interest to participate at every stage. As well, attempts at consultation in this study did not always elicit much feedback; many participants had other aspects of organization and activism or family and illness concerns taking up most of their time. The group leaders and the research team and I had several frank discussions about our similar and differing priorities, skills, and interests. As noted in the summary table (see table 8, page 140), we have found other ways to work together.
4 All participant names are pseudonyms.
5 See Sinding et al., chapter 6, this volume, for discussion of mainstream cancer support groups' failure to address lesbians' support needs. A common reason given by groups, the authors note, is that it is 'not their mandate' to address diversity issues.

REFERENCES

Abrums, M.E., & Leppa, C. (2001). Beyond cultural competence: Teaching about race, gender, class and sexual orientation. *Journal of Nursing Education, 40*(6), 270–6.

Altman, R. (1996). *Waking up/fighting back: The politics of breast cancer.* Boston: Little, Brown.

Berlin, A., Johansson, S.E., & Törnkvist, L. (2006). Working conditions and cultural competence when interacting with children and parents of foreign origin: Primary Child Health Nurses' opinions. *Scandinavian Journal of Caring Sciences, 20*(2), 160–8.

Betancourt, J.R., Green, A.R., Carrillo, J.E., & Ananeh-Firempong, O. (2003). Defining cultural competence: A practical framework for addressing racial/ethnic disparities in health and health care. *Public Health Reports, 118*(4), 293.

Bhopal, R. (1998). Spectre of racism in health and health care: Lessons from history and the United States. *British Medical Journal, 316*(7149), 1970–3.

Bourjolly, J.N., Barg, F.K., & Hirschman, K.B. (2003). African-American and white women's appraisal of their breast cancer. *Journal of Psychosocial Oncology, 21*(3), 43–61.

Burman, E., Smailes, S.L., & Chantler, K. (2004). 'Culture' as a barrier to service provision and delivery: Domestic violence services for minoritized women. *Critical Social Policy, 24*, 332–57.

Bussema, E., & Nemec, P. (2006). Training to increase cultural competence. *Psychiatric Rehabilitation Journal, 30*(1), 71–3.

Carter, B. (2000). *Realism and racism: Concepts of race in sociological research.* London: Routledge.

Collins, P.H. (1990). *Black feminist thought: Knowledge, consciousness, and the politics of empowerment.* Boston: Unwin Hyman.

Davies, B. (1997). The subject of post-structuralism: A reply to Alison Jones. *Gender and Education, 9*(3), 271–83.

Davis, P.C., & Rankin, L.L. (2006). Guidelines for making existing health education programs more culturally appropriate. *American Journal of Health Education, 37*(4), 250–2.

Dennis, G.C. (2001). Racism in medicine: Planning for the future. *Journal of the National Medical Association, 93*(3 Suppl.), 1–5.

Doutrich, D., & Storey, M. (2006). Cultural competence and organizational change: Lasting results of an institutional linkage. *Home Health Care Management & Practice, 18*(5), 356–60.

Eliason, M.J. (1999). Nursing's role in racism and African American women's health. *Health Care for Women International, 20*, 209–19.

Essed, P. (1991). Understanding everyday racism: An interdisciplinary theory. In John H. Stanfield II (Ed.), *Sage series on race and ethnic relations.* Newbury Park: Sage.

Fassin, D. (2001). Culturalism as ideology. In C.M. Obermeyer (Ed.), *Cultural perspectives on reproductive health* (pp. 300–17). Oxford University Press.

Fellows, M.L., & Razack, S.H. (1998). The race to innocence: Confronting hierarchical relations among women. *Journal of Gender, Race and Justice, 1*(2), 335–52.

Fine, M., Weis, L., Weseen, S., & Wong, L. (2003). For whom? Qualitative research, representations, and social responsibilities. In N.K. Denzin & Y.S. Lincoln (Eds.), *The landscape of qualitative research: Theories and issues.* Thousand Oaks, CA: Sage Publications.

Foucault, M. (1972). *The archeology of knowledge and the discourse of language.* New York: Pantheon.

Foucault, M. (1980). Truth and power. In C. Gordon (Ed.), *Power/knowledge: Selected interviews and other writings, 1972–1977.* New York: Pantheon Books.

Foucault, M. (1984). What is an author? In P. Rabinow (Ed.), *The Foucault reader.* New York: Pantheon.

Fowers, B.J., & Davidov, B.J. (2006). The virtue of multiculturalism: Personal transformation, character, and openness to the other. *American Psychologist, 61*, 581–94.

Francis, C.K. (2001). Medical ethos and social responsibility in clinical medicine. *Journal of Urban Health, 78*(1), 29–45.

Galambos, C.M. (2003). Moving cultural diversity toward cultural competence in health care. *Health & Social Work, 28*(1), 3–22.

Gamble, V.N. (1997). Under the shadow of Tuskegee: African Americans and health care. *American Journal of Public Health, 87*, 1773–8.

Gilroy, P. (1987). Conclusion: Urban social movements, 'race,' and community. In P. Gilroy (Ed.), *'There ain't no black in the Union Jack': The cultural politics of race and nation* (pp. 223–50). London: Hutchinson.

Glenn, E.N. (1992). From servitude to service work: Historical continuities in the racial division of paid reproductive labour. *Signs, 18*(1), 1–43.

Goldberg, D.T. (1993). *Racist culture, philosophy and the politics of meaning.* Oxford: Blackwell.

Guidry, J.J., Matthews-Juarez, P., & Copeland, V.A. (2003). Barriers to breast cancer control for African-American women: The interdependence of culture and psychosocial issues. *Cancer, 97*(S1), 318–23.

Gunaratnam, Y. (1997). Culture is not enough: A critique of multi-culturalism in palliative care. In D. Field, J. Hockey, and N. Small (Eds.), *Death, gender and ethnicity* (pp. 166–86). London: Routledge.

Hall, S. (1997). The work of representation. In S. Hall (Ed.), *Representation: Cultural representations and signifying practices* (pp. 15–64). London: Sage Publications.

Harrison, J., MacGibbon, L., & Morton, M. (2001). Regimes of trustworthiness in qualitative research: The rigors of reciprocity. *Qualitative Inquiry, 7*(3), 323–45.

Harrison, R.W. (2001). Impact of biomedical research on African Americans. *Journal of the National Medical Association, 93*(S3), 6–7.

166   Cancer on the Margins

Higginbotham, E.B. (1992). African-American women's history and the meta-language of race. *Signs, 17*(2), 264.

Jackson, J.C., Taylor, V.M., Chitnarong, K., Mahloch, J., Fischer, M., Sam, R., & Seng, P. (2000). Development of a cervical cancer control intervention program for Cambodian American women. *Journal of Community Health, 25,* 359–75.

Jeffery, D., & Nelson, J. (2008). Racing to culture: a critical race analysis of culturalist approaches in social work and health settings. Unpublished manuscript.

Jørgenson, M., & Phillips, L. (2002). *Discourse analysis as theory and method.* Thousand Oaks and London: Sage.

Kendall, G., & Wickham, G. (1999). *Using Foucault's methods.* London: Sage.

Kinney, A.Y., Emery, G., Dudley, W., & Croyle, R. (2002). Screening behaviors among African American women at high risk of breast cancer: Do beliefs about God matter? *Oncology Nursing Forum, 29,* 835–43.

Kofman, E. (2004). Gendered global migrations. *International Feminist Journal of Politics, 6,* 643–65.

Lannin, D.R., Mathews, H.F., Mitchell, J., & Swanson, M.S. (2002). Impacting cultural attitudes in African-American women to decrease breast cancer mortality. *American Journal of Surgery, 184,* 418–23.

Lather, P. (1988). Feminist perspectives on empowering research methodologies. *Women's Studies International Forum, 11,* 569–81.

Leigh, J.W. (1998). *Communicating for cultural competence.* Toronto: Allyn & Bacon.

Mays, N., & Pope, C. (1995). Qualitative research: Rigour and qualitative research. *British Medical Journal, 311*(8), 109–12.

McClintock, A. (1995). *Imperial leather: Race, gender and sexuality in the colonial contest.* New York: Routledge.

McKennis, A.T. (1999). Caring for the Islamic patient. *Association of Operating Room Nurses Journal, 69,* 1185–206.

Mir, G., & Tovey, P. (2002). Cultural competency: Professional action and South Asian carers. *Journal of Management in Medicine, 16,* 7–19.

Nairn, S., et al. (2004). Multicultural or anti-racist teaching in nurse education: A critical appraisal. *Nurse Education Today, 24*(3), 188–95.

Nelson, J., & Agyapong, F. (2004). Women of colour living with breast cancer: Exploring the search for support. *Canadian Woman Studies,* Fall, 167–72.

Park, Y. (2005). Culture as deficit: A critical discourse analysis of the concept of culture in contemporary social work discourse. *Journal of Sociology and Social Welfare 32*(3), 11–33.

Parreñas, R.S. (2001). Servants of globalization. Stanford University Press.

Phillips, J.M., Cohen, M.Z., & Tarzian, A.J. (2001). African American women's experiences with breast cancer screening. *Journal of Nursing Scholarship,* 33(2), 135–40.

Popkewitz, T.S. (1998). *Struggling for the soul: The politics of schooling and the construction of the teacher.* New York: Teacher's College Press.

Raso, R. (2006). Cultural competence: Integral in diverse populations. *Nursing Management, 37*(7), 56.

Razack, S. (1995). The perils of talking about culture: Schooling research on South and East Asian students. *Race, Gender and Class, 2*(3), 67–82.

Razack, S. (1998). *Looking white people in the eye: Gender, race, and culture in courtrooms and classrooms.* University of Toronto Press.

Razack, S. (Ed.). (2002). *Race, space and the law: Unmapping a white settler society.* Toronto: Between the Lines Press.

Shen, M.Z. (2004). Cultural competence models in nursing: A selected annotated bibliography. *Journal of Transcultural Nursing, 15*(4), 317–22.

Taylor, J. (1999). Colonizing images and diagnostic labels: Oppressive mechanisms for African American women's health. *Advances in Nursing Science, 21*(3), 32–45.

Thapar-Björkert, S., & Henry, M. (2004). Reassessing the research relationship: Location, position and power in fieldwork accounts. *Social Research Methodology, 7,* 363–81.

Todd, J., & Baldwin, C.M. (2006). Palliative care and culture: An optimistic view. *Journal of Multicultural Nursing Health, 12*(2), 28–32.

van Dijk, T.A. (1993). Elite discourse and racism. In John H. Stanfield II (Ed.), *Sage series on race and ethnic relations* (vol. 6). Newbury Park: Sage.

Watts, R.J. (2003). Race consciousness and the health of African Americans. *Online Journal of Issues in Nursing, 8*(1), http://nursingworld.org/ojin/topic20/tpc_3.htm

Waxler, N.M. (1990). Introduction. In *Cross cultural caring: A handbook in Western Canada.* Vancouver: UBC Press.

Westby, D.L. (1991). *The growth of sociological theory: Human nature, knowledge and social change.* Englewood Cliffs, NJ: Prentice-Hall.

White, D.G. (1985). *Ar'n't I a woman?: Female slaves in the plantation south.* New York: W.W. Norton.

Xu, Y., Shelton, D., Polifroni, E.C., & Anderson, E. (2006). Advances in conceptualization of cultural care and cultural competence in nursing: An initial assessment. *Home Health Care Management & Practice, 18,* 386–93.

Yee, J., & Dumbrill, G. (2003). Whiteout: Looking for race in Canadian social work practice. In A. Al-Krenawi and J. Graham (Eds.), *Multicultural social work in Canada: Working with diverse ethno-racial communities* (pp. 98–121). Don Mills: Oxford University Press.

PART FOUR

Reflections on Research:
From Different Standpoints

8 Reflections from an Intersection: Identity, History, Cancer, and Social Change

JENNIFER J. NELSON AND JUDY GOULD

> I wonder ... what can't I see in the transcripts, given where I'm coming from?
>
> –Judy

Introduction to an Intersection

This chapter is written from the intersection of several stories. One involves that of two researchers thinking through personal histories that have led us to work with women who have breast cancer. Another story is that of grappling with our positions – socially, economically, professionally, and personally – vis-à-vis the research participants with whom we work. Another is that of our participants' struggles to resolve their information and support needs following a diagnosis of breast cancer, across profound barriers of race, culture, and low-income status. Yet another story involves our relationship to the data we collect – how to 'read' or analyse it, and how to best disseminate and utilize it in the service of social change that will eventually benefit women in the communities with whom we work. When we reflect on processes of change, then, we are concerned both with external change, through the transformative potential of research-based knowledge, and with how internal change, through personal reflection, influences the quality and direction of our research.

We find ourselves standing at this curious intersection time and time again. We are social scientists doing qualitative work in the health-care field, which is almost entirely biomedically and quantitatively informed. We are trained in the fields of social and community psychology (Judy) and sociology of education (Jennifer) with a strong focus on issues of social justice and equity. We have a mandate to work with socially and economically marginalized women in an environment in which their particular needs are only beginning to be recognized. We often employ community-based research methods in a field where listening to patients' perspectives is a relatively new concept. Yet, while we often find ourselves on the margins in the contexts of the health-care research world and politics, we are outsiders to many of our target communities.

We are both white, young, well-educated, and recently upper-middle class women; our job is to carry out research that will positively affect the lives of women who are low-income and women of colour, who are middle age on average, and who have breast cancer. While the populations with whom we tend to work have lower breast cancer incidence rates than white, middle-class, or affluent women, their mortality rates are higher. They also face particular economic and social barriers to care, support, and information.

Jennifer's pilot work with women of colour (see table 8, page 140) has been two-fold, aiming on the one hand to hear and document the concerns of the women, and, more broadly, beginning to develop a systemic analysis of how racism can impact women's ability to find support and information that meet their needs (Nelson & Agyapong, 2004). Judy has explored the financial issues and concerns of individual lower-income Canadian women with breast cancer (see table 4, page 76). This study is the first in a research program where she is endeavouring to understand the systemic/political barriers to affordable cancer care (Gould, 2004).

To do this work, we must routinely form research relationships that are mired in social power differentials. We cross historically entrenched boundaries to work with populations that have been colonized, exploited, and monitored by dominant races and classes – not to mention over-researched, but rarely with equity as the end goal. Informed by feminist and auto-ethnographic traditions (see Ellis & Bochner, 2000; Church, 1995), we believe that personal reflection is essential to responsible research and analysis. Our disciplinary fields in the social sciences have seen the harm wrought by years of uncritical 'objective' approaches to research in which already-subjugated populations are treated as informants at best and guinea pigs at worst by researchers who feel entitled to probe their lives, publish data that remain within elite intellectual circles, and leave without a trace (Hagey, 1997).

We have studied the effects of knowledge production that is uninformed by critical reflection about power and social marginality (Nelson, 2008a, 2008b). Such knowledge – such stories – underpin policy, law, healthcare, education, and government. In other words, the stories that we produce about groups or individuals have implications for what happens to those groups or individuals in their everyday lives. The way in which we produce stories is undeniably influenced by our own gaze, our standpoint, the history we bring to a research moment. Social positionality, standpoint theory (Harding, 1991; Stoetzler & Yuval-Davis, 2002), situated knowing (Haraway, 1991), and 'sociology of knowledge' (Smith, 1990) are just a few examples of theories from a wide body of social thought that has incited many researchers to analyse and articulate the problems of location, subjectivity, and power with regard to knowledge production. The study of the social aspects of health presents no exception to these difficult and political processes. In many ways, we have found that issues of social equity are still considered relatively new and novel within healthcare fields. Researchers are just beginning to be aware of power dynamics and different service needs among diverse populations, and are only recently noting that systemic discrimination is a key barrier for many ill people when accessing care and support (Malat, 2006).

We have a responsibility to learn from mistakes of the past and to remain attentive to our personal investments and professional decisions in doing this work. Moreover, critique of the problematics of unequal research relationships must be ongoing. It evolves with the researcher, the research relationship, the particular project, and with reflection over time. What we point to in this chapter, then, are not finite processes or conclusive 'recipes' to avoid the pitfalls of power imbalances in research but, rather, some particular issues that have been key for us. What we consider to be beneficial experiences of change are those ways in which our research approaches and processes have been challenged, enriched, and transformed through critical reflection, including, more recently, within the conversations we present here.

Wanting to explore some of these issues in the context of our current roles, we decided to hold four recorded conversations in which we 'interviewed' each other regarding our views, social positions, and the challenges we face in our work. This chapter focuses on several aspects of our dialogue, namely, those raised by the following questions:

• How do our personal life experiences influence our project choices?
• What aspects of the work attract us? What aspects do we resist?

- How do our subject positions – the situations in which we find ourselves with regard to systems of power, privilege, dominance, and marginality – change over time? How does this influence our research?
- As researchers working for social change and to improve the experiences of marginalized women, what are our reflections about the political nature of this work?

Following our conversations, we took notes from the recordings, transcribed excerpts of dialogue, and distilled the results into several key issues. Much of our discussion fell in and around two themes:

1 Subjectivity or Subject Position: With these terms, we refer to the interlinked aspects of our identities that shape the ways in which we negotiate power relations, whether as privileged or disadvantaged, depending on the situation or context. Subjectivity is not fixed, but is constituted in relationship to others and to social and political processes over time (Foucault, 1982). Facets of identity that we discussed included race, class, gender, cultural capital, and personal histories as they influence our work.

2 Social Change: This part of our discussion centred on the accountabilities and responsibilities we feel around doing work that has social change as its end goal. It included attention to the processes of entering and exiting the work, the role of the researcher, and our concerns about the multiple meanings and expectations surrounding 'change' itself.

In the following sections we will explore our research questions and themes using portions of our dialogues (which are prefaced with the speaker's name). We also illustrate particular points using quotes provided to us by the women who participated in our respective research projects (Nelson & Agyapong, 2004; Gould, 2004).

Reviewing Social Positions: A Tale of Two Subjects

We began our interviews with each other by reviewing some central aspects of identity that we have to consider in our work, attending to both our backgrounds and where we find ourselves today. Although we told different stories of class background, we both spoke about our experiences of unease around the shifting of class identity that occurs with growing educational and professional status.

Coming from a white working-class background, Jennifer talked about class signifiers that served as both real and perceived barriers when pursuing higher education. This experience was informed by her move from a rural area to a major urban centre, and her entrée into an elite university music program. At the same time, she notes in the dialogue that she lacked class consciousness while experiencing this sense of 'not fitting.'

JENNIFER: The university was an alienating world for me – I felt that other people there seemed to have a sense of entitlement, as if they'd always just been expected to go. In the music program, when I first met my piano instructor, he asked 'who have you studied with?' and I thought – 'how would he ever know the person (from 1,500 km away) – like, why would you ask that?!' But people really expected you to have studied with someone who was 'known.' It was considered bizarre that I'd never seen an opera. It was equally appalling that I only spoke one language … So you quickly got a sense of 'should I even be here?' – although at that time I didn't really have an analysis, and wouldn't have used Bourdieu's term 'cultural capital'[1] – which I find quite useful now in thinking about privilege.

A later academic focus on racism and white privilege further complicated her ideas about class differences within a racially dominant group and how she was situated in the circles of higher education.

JENNIFER: In my work I've had to think a lot about how whites in dominant positions in our social context – North America – produce knowledge about marginal, racialized groups and marginalized communities. I've focused on the impact that knowledge has in people's lives. I have traced the history of settlement in my home province with regard to race and where various groups ended up, and the relative material privilege of my own ancestors as they settled in Nova Scotia.

At the same time, as I've thought more about my own life, I realize that privilege was in some ways mitigated by a working-class background. Women of colour in the university would sometimes make statements directed toward white women beginning with things like 'Elite women like you' ... I understood and accepted where this was coming from, but I couldn't relate to the term 'elite' – it didn't reflect my experience: I couldn't help thinking that my father came home with dirt under his fingernails, that my mother never set foot in an airplane until she was 47 years old ... So I didn't know how to respond to those comments because I knew that to be defensive about it would be taken as an attempt to obscure my white privilege.

Queried by Judy, Jennifer reflected on how her class position changed as a result of negotiating those conundrums to gain an education, and that her current position represents something of a surprising shift:

JENNIFER: I often feel like I'm just 'passing' as 'a professional,' but I know that to my research participants it doesn't show that I come from working-class middle-of-nowhere – and in some ways it might not matter, since whiteness is likely the biggest and more immediate difference they notice, and we have talked about that together. But I feel some irony in the fact that it is only now that I have a more developed class and race analysis and an education around equity issues that I'm in a much higher socioeconomic bracket.

Judy's story began differently, took a series of different turns, and led us to an important dialogue about entitlement and privilege.

JUDY: When I engaged in the work with low-income women it was important for me to be connected to them somehow, even if that connection had to be dredged up from the past. My mother and father divorced when I was 14 years old. My mother, sisters and I went from middle class to living below the poverty line. Even still, my sisters and I were 'entitled' to hold fast to our cultural capital. We never questioned that we were going to go to university though my mother and father could contribute nothing financially. And I've always felt that I could access any resource. I had no idea then of the white and classed undergirding of my resourcefulness.

Recognizing that Judy had cultural capital but no money to support her taken-for-granted future and that Jennifer was financially sound but lacked cultural capital, we discussed how 'class' signifies more than just money. It also entails culture, knowledge, social signifiers, and status. In this light, we discussed the racialized and classed ability to maintain a 'toehold on respectability' (Fellows & Razack, 1998). This refers to the ways in which we are able to mobilize aspects of our subject positions that allow access to the professions, acquisitions, and values that embody white, middle-class notions of respectability.

In particular, we discussed some ways in which subjectivity influences our research, our relationships to participants, and the analysis we bring to the work. For instance, in working with participants from lower-income communities, it is helpful to have a more nuanced understanding of class privilege as more than simply money or income, and to recognize the fluidity of poverty and its interconnections with other institutionalized forms of domination. Personal experience can enrich that understanding when read alongside theoretical analysis. At the same time, we cannot assume that having a similar experience enables one to relate better to another; no matter where we come from, researchers need to recognize how we're differently positioned within social hierarchies. We need to think about the ways in which our own positions might enable us to overlook – or never see – angles of the analysis we're embarking on.

What Can't I See in the Research? Literal and Figurative Mirrors

Judy's opening query, 'What can't I see?' captures the essence of a dilemma we both face in our research: How does where we come from affect our relationship with participants across social differences? Can it be possible to 'know what we don't know,' to predict when our subject positions are acting as blind spots? To a large degree, we approach these issues by attempting to make our subject positions, the interpretive process, and our resulting analysis as transparent as we can. But what does this look like, when subject positions – our own and others' – are dynamic and complex, rather than straightforward or fixed? (Heron, 2005). Yasmin Gunaratnam, writing about research on ethnicity and race, reminds us of a necessary fluidity in how we describe and work with difference and subjectivity:

> while there must be temporary moments of closure in the defining of racial and ethnic categories in order to do research, these points of closure must also be opened up again in the process of doing research and in analysis. They must be opened up in ways that enable us to look at and hear how 'race' and ethnicity are given situated meaning within accounts, and how

meanings can be both secured and made more ambiguous and uncertain. (2003, p. 38)

Lila Abu-Lughod (1991) encourages researchers to pay attention to the *particulars* of participant's lives – the concrete moments and stories in which conflict, power, and resistance often figure. We were curious about what would happen if we flipped this around and thought about the particulars of our own lives as we engaged in research. As with Jennifer's experience of negotiating expectations in the music program, we reflect on these moments as signifiers of disruptions, or 'openings' in which we must look at the differently situated meanings of identities and power:

JUDY: I noticed that as I began this work, when getting ready for interviews I would choose to wear more casual clothing, would choose not to wear jewellery. I noticed I wanted to appear demure – to try to pass into whatever 'culture' I felt I was stepping into – assuming there existed only one 'other.'

I was also aware that the low-income women on my advisory committee would speak up at meetings but would often preface their remarks with 'I don't have the right words like all of you guys' … I realized that the signifiers of dress and talk – the processes and moments of disruption – are the passageways to revealing hegemonic power relations. These moments are stored in the particularities, in everyday life.

JENNIFER: It's also interesting how context-dependent these things are. My assumption also used to be that I should dress down, to avoid alienating people. Then during graduate school my supervisor, a woman of colour, once talked about the politics of race and dress. She noted that white people could come to a meeting in jeans, but people of colour could never do the same. I can't believe how naïve I was about this now that I go to events with women of colour in the community – for one thing, I could never hope to dress as well as they do! [laughter] I fear it would be seen as disrespectful to be too casual, and I am probably extra aware of that as an outsider to the community. But more importantly, I hadn't thought of it as an expression of privilege to dress down in some contexts, to be 'at home' enough in a certain place that you don't have to think about establishing respectability or commanding respect, and to be assured that no one else will question your entitlement to be there. So there is yet another particularity, another class and race signifier that is not what we might expect, given where we're coming from.

Recalling Gunaratnam's caution, we want to be clear that there are no 'rules' to be uncovered or correct formulas that can be figured out and applied; for example, finding out about cultural norms and copying them in order to 'fit in' is neither possible nor desirable. That kind of approach evokes an essentialist understanding of differences and similarities – one that, we realized, is often easy to fall into as researchers from relatively privileged positions. Rather, by noticing what might appear to be small things, and paying attention to our discomfort, we gain insight into the power imbalances that underlie and inform our work.

The point is not to learn to dress differently or say the right thing, but to take these relatively unimportant things as signals to ask ourselves, for example, how am I thinking about this difference? What is my discomfort and how is it produced? How might that affect my view of and interaction with my participants? What are the sets of relations, historically and socially, that inform how I encounter these participants and what our relationship will entail (see Brah, 1996; Lewis, 2000)? The small signifiers, upon reflection, have the potential to lead us out of the 'individualized' moment of the one-on-one interview and towards a more critically informed and historically situated view of relationships and the operation of power.

These questions can be mobilized as part of our analytic framework – so that the research 'problem' is rooted in particular socioeconomic systems and relationships. Further, the research 'solution' – for example, how to make services more accessible to women living in poverty – is more likely to be informed by an understanding of how poverty is lived, what the root causes are, and how researchers, care providers, and participants/patients might then go about addressing some systemic barriers rather than treating individual disadvantages as aberrations.

Does Cancer Have a Colour? The Quagmire of Analysis

So if we are predisposed to be blindsided by aspects of our subject positions, what do we make of others' stories? What can't we see in our research transcripts? How do we listen with empathy and with both an ear and an eye to difference? When we interpret another person's words, what is important to think about? Perhaps most importantly, how can we be aware of what we don't know?

As qualitative social scientists, dealing with the social world and people's complex identities and lives, we necessarily question and overturn traditional notions of truth in favour of more situated and subjective understandings of reality (Haraway, 1991; Flax, 1990). We must operate with the assumption that 'knowledge' is produced and productive, that what we are hearing from research subjects is shaped by their own identities and histories as well as our own, and by the relationships we form with our participants.

Foucault's conceptualization of power is useful here, as it encompasses the multi-directional flow of power relations. His theory centrally acknowledges that power does not simply operate one way, from the top down, and there is always resistance and deliberation among those who are subjugated (Foucault, 1980). In this sense, we also know that subjectivities and the power they embody can affect what participants feel comfortable talking about, how they will shape their responses to us. And by the same token, we cannot assume that similarity or shared identity necessarily leads to a 'truer' or more open revelation of experience (see Allen & Cloyes, 2005; Gunaratnam, 2003, chap. 4).

We are not, then, uncovering people's 'real' thoughts or experiences per se; we are finding out how people understand, interpret, and narrate their experiences in a particular context, in light of the current time and place and research relationship. 'Truth' is co-constructed in our conversation, in the case of interviews, and is informed by our experiences and knowledge in these and other kinds of research work. This doesn't make it less valid; rather, it acknowledges that external factors, who we are as people and what we think we are doing as researchers, shape the interactions through which data is created and analysed.

In the following exchange, we discuss our experiences around finding out about power relations through interviews and the kinds of dilemmas we have faced when trying to analyse how participants talked about such relations:

JENNIFER: How did discussions about poverty itself play out in your interviews with the women?
JUDY: Participants tended to talk about how proud they were of what little money they had, or how far they managed to make the money stretch. Most women didn't provide a systemic analysis around poverty and cancer. They describe individual circumstances and how they coped. One group of women invited me to dinner following the focus group that was held with them. At dinner they

asked 'what did you find during the study that you were surprised about?' I said that I'd expected them to be angrier, more politicized around the impact of their situations, more upset with 'the system,' but they replied 'we're embarrassed' (about their low-income status). So the stigma attached to poverty made it difficult for them to talk openly.

JENNIFER: It is difficult to get at. When I was writing my dissertation I read another study that had been done in the same community on which my own research was focused, and the researchers' questionnaire had questions like 'Do you consider yourself to be poor?'! It was appalling. I thought, 'How can you ask a question like that in such a stark way and take all the answers at face value? And how can you ask that as a white academic with money, going into a poor, black community?!'

JUDY: Again, it is in the particularities and moments of people's stories that the reality of poverty is revealed. For the most part, my participants stressed positive things, like the few services that had been available to them. But then they would talk about walking home for 45 minutes after their chemotherapy, or not being able to afford to eat at the hospital while they waited for their blood work or for a delayed chemotherapy treatment. One participant had a more critical perspective on the system as a whole, but I really noticed the lack of a discourse of 'entitlement.'

JENNIFER: I struggle with that kind of thing ... I have a specific dilemma right now: I believe that a great deal of racism is coming out in the stories I hear from women of colour, but only a few of them actually name racism. They are more likely to say that a problem is 'not about race' but about something else. They will say 'cancer has no colour' – which is true – suggesting that everyone deserves equal treatment, but I still see colour as making a big difference in the services they receive, or even in what they feel comfortable accessing. Also, a lot of women will say there is no racism, but then later in the interview disavow it indirectly. For example, they'll say, 'I just feel more comfortable around other black women,' or 'There are things we can't talk about if there are white people in the support group.' Or they will say, 'the problem isn't about racism, it's about the secrecy in our community about cancer, how we can't talk about it.' To me, all those things are part of larger systemic and historical issues of racism.

In community-based work, actually in any research, a major ethical principle is that you follow participants' words and stay as 'true' as possible to their views. I can't put words in their mouths, but at the same time I sometimes disagree when they say a particular problem isn't about racism. I want to be able to say that while cancer has no colour, coping with it does. Being white, working with non-white women, adds another layer to that – for a white woman to say she sees racism where participants of colour do not, can be a further expression of power.[2]

JUDY: I know what you mean. I think about the same things, and just recently I am starting to feel that it's okay to write and wonder about participants' seeming lack of 'entitlement' as my own observation. I check back with them to assure their words and meanings are intact and that I'm not reading into it something they didn't mean to say, but I think it is okay to have a different, albeit privileged, interpretation.

JENNIFER: That's true. But as you mentioned, our analysis does hold more weight – researchers' voices will tend to be heard and valued more. My voice – not only as a researcher with credentials, but as a white person – will be heard above those of racialized or poor women who have historically been assumed incapable of representing themselves.

In thinking through this issue, we returned to the useful concept of a 'toehold' on respectability. We became aware that our *raison d'être* is to interpret oppressive experiences of our participants in order to increase responsiveness to those issues within the cancer care system. Poor and racialized women may not have the same opportunities to do so. For these women, to 'come out' as political often means a loss of some of this toehold – it might bring about more hardship; those in dominant positions may perceive it as 'angry' or 'radical' – characteristics particularly scorned by the dominant group. 'Outing' oneself as a political activist places one further on the margins when one is already there, struggling to survive. In the cases of our participants, we discussed the possibility of their need to disavow negative aspects of their social location in order to retain a toehold on respectability, particularly in light of the complicated emotions around living with racialized and classed stigma.

Michelle Fine and her colleagues (2000) discuss the issue of 'trading' on racial and class privilege in order to bring the issues facing marginalized people to policy makers and the public. In a similar sense, we talked about how community-based research sometimes affords us chances to create spaces in which marginalized women can better represent themselves (for example, by helping raise awareness of the issues, referring the media to speak to the groups we work with, setting up meetings with policy makers in which patients can participate, using the research to support funding proposals for community-run projects and programs). Although it is not straightforward, collaborative work has the potential to at least partially mitigate the dynamic of 'researcher as expert.'

'The Elephant in the Room': Unsexy Content as Bread and Butter

Nobody ever ask me anything, none of the doctors, nurses, none of them ever asked me how you get home when you take your treatment, you know what I mean? ... I'm not looked upon you see, I am below their notice ... They figure ... why would I want to help her, who is she? ... I mean you want to help people, you help everybody.

–Research Participant, Judy's lower-income women
with breast cancer study

One of the problems is that many people of colour find in hospitals and different places where they go to get treatment, they are sort of treated differently. They don't treat them the same as they treat Caucasians, the other groups ... we are the same and we like to be treated with respect, dignity, as other nationalities.

–Research Participant, Jennifer's women of colour
with breast cancer study

The participants quoted here speak of concrete disparities in their health service experiences. Such examples are abundant in our work, encompassing a realm of issues that are often difficult to bring to the attention of healthcare professionals and policy makers:

JUDY: When I started at this research unit and became engaged in my first research topic about low-income women with breast cancer, I felt like 'poverty isn't sexy' as a topic for research. It's the elephant in the room, the issue people in dominant institutions want swept off the agenda.

JENNIFER: A difficult thing about working toward equity in institutions not traditionally geared toward it is that, unlike teaching graduate classes, there often is not a good or obvious starting point. Students choose to go to university; and particularly in graduate school, you can assume to some degree that people are there because they have some interest in learning about what you're teaching. In the hospital, examining inequities is not the reason anyone's there – we're asking them to look at issues they didn't choose to look at, or that were not a consideration in their career choice. That's not to say it's everyone – some people are interested and supportive of our work – but there is also bound to be a lot of resistance and a feeling that these issues don't 'fit' with the rest of the work in healthcare (even though there is plenty of research demonstrating how poverty and racism negatively affect health). Remember – at both of the psychosocial oncology conferences we went to last year, there was practically no attention to diverse experiences or issues of oppression?

JUDY: – And how disappointing since at one conference, the theme was 'Understanding Diversities – development of strategies for psychosocial oncology'!

Institutional change is both broad and individual – it requires individuals in decision-making positions to examine their own subjectivities as much as we have begun to suggest here. This is not comfortable, not reflective of the liberal concept most of us would like to have of ourselves as fair, equitable, and non-discriminatory. These issues often feel 'new' in health settings, while they were commonplace in our previous academic training and community work.

JUDY: It's also easy to get confused between the pressure to make the cancer experience itself better and the social justice bent of our research unit. Since we operate in a healthcare setting, at a major cancer centre, psychosocial work is held up against stem cell research, new chemotherapy techniques, and the identification of tumour markers – again, sexy topics! [laughter] It is easy to feel that we're not able to enact the kind of change that is fundamental to illness, that we can't enact any change fast enough, and that our role is seen as less important.

JENNIFER: I think we have both often experienced healthcare as a strange and somewhat alienating setting, coming from social science backgrounds. But I've realized in discussing this that it's important to remind ourselves that the work 'matters' in a very different way. It is about equity and access to services. 'Social justice' work could really be done at any site in some capacity – for us, it's almost like it 'happens' to be in cancer.

JUDY: Right. While people probably expect that cancer is our central 'topic' of work, our entry points are actually from the perspectives of equity – feminism, social justice, anti-racism and so forth. I've often thought, 'like cancer isn't bad enough on its own, we're dealing with poverty and racism too ...'

JENNIFER: I know. And sometimes I feel some guilt around the fact that I'm really benefiting from these stories from women of colour about their struggles and hardships. We can focus on issues that are of interest to us – and be paid for it; these issues are our bread and butter – while participants are, at the end of the day, still living with critical illness and everything else. We have some choice and some reprieve.

JUDY: And there is some irony in the fact that we draw on relatively privileged positions in order to try to change things for others. As we discussed before, our voices, our analyses, will hold more weight than others'. You never escape that difference; even with our attempts to make projects very participatory and incorporate communities, you are forced to mobilize around your status to make anything better for anyone.

This brought our discussion around to the issue of what constitutes 'change,' our responsibility to our participants for making sure the research 'makes a difference,' and our sense of the researcher's role.

Social Change: The Tyranny of the Shelf

The only thing I will be a little bit sad about is if this does not go anywhere, if all of this is done and we see nothing come out of it, we see it going on the shelves where ... [there is] quite a stack stacked on shelves already, gathering dust, nothing being done ... and you know I would like something, somebody to pay attention to this and put some action into it. That will really make me very happy and I could think that my trip down [here] will not be for nothing, but something.

–Research Participant, Jennifer's women of colour
with breast cancer study

During one of our dialogues, Jennifer described to Judy how she'd felt a knot in her stomach upon hearing the above participant's words. She noted the sense of pressure that it induced, even though she was aware that she and this participant were 'on the same side.' In our focus on community-based participatory research, we frequently hear and think about the expectations of our participants, and often with reference to their past experiences with research that did not 'go anywhere.' We feel responsible for seeing that research has some transformative potential, while also balancing the fact that change takes time, and much is not within our immediate capacity to control – for instance, funding decisions, policy making, entrenched institutional practices, not to mention the time required for research itself.

Even though research dissemination is a fundamental component of all our projects, we sometimes question how change can be not only made, but measured. The assessment of impact is an important component of our work – for us, but also to funders, participants, and other stakeholders. Almost always, the concern is expressed using the same exact words – referring to the proverbial 'shelf' upon which 'bad' researchers will inevitably leave their work. At one point, Jennifer expressed to Judy, 'I'm so tired of hearing about the damn shelf!'

JUDY: I felt a real resistance to getting into the work at first because it seemed too big a problem, like I had no power to make anything change. Even mobilizing people around the study felt overwhelming. It made me feel incompetent when the effect of the project wasn't far-reaching and really public. It's easier when working with an already connected community, like in the lesbian community (where our colleague does research). 'Low-income' isn't an identity, it's a stigma – and many women cycle in and out of poverty. So, what does social change look like?

JENNIFER: I had resistance too. Partly it was around getting in 'too deep': I wasn't clear – am still not totally clear – on when my role ended. And these issues are huge and ongoing – equal access to emotional and practical support for cancer diagnosis, treatment and aftercare; they really don't have a logical or obvious end. The issues we're interested in are systemic in nature – they are about racism and socioeconomic discrimination – they aren't going to go anywhere in a hurry. I'm in this kind of work for the long haul, but it must be done through a variety of projects over time, as part of a bigger research program and in conjunction with many other researchers and communities. So I feared the possible expectation that this project in itself would make a big difference in people's lives right away, and that if it wasn't seen to do 'enough,' that criticism would be tied to the troubled history of white researchers taking advantage of communities of colour as 'data' but then not giving anything back to the community. There's a whole history that is implicitly referenced when we make decisions about how involved we become, and what our responsibilities are. It isn't just about practical considerations, like how much time we have at the moment.

Our concerns over the lack of clarity around 'entering and exiting' the work seem endemic to participatory research on a practical level, but in light of our earlier considerations about 'doing the right thing' (expressed in those small examples like dress and talk), we also wondered if there is something more going on. Fears around being the 'bad' researcher, or failing to improve things, are also about subjectivity. Here, we balance the accountability for doing applicable and useful work with the knowledge that 'helping' is also a historically-laden concept that has been central to colonial projects and founded on dramatic power imbalances (Heron, 2007; Jeffery, 2002). How do we acknowledge power differences without overstating them in such a way that inequality is even more deeply entrenched? The collaborative nature of the work figured centrally as we thought through this balance between doing accountable, applicable work, and recognizing some of the boundaries around responsibility.

During this part of the discussion, Judy reflected on the important aspect that the process of community-based participatory action research (CBPAR) takes some of the pressure off *her alone* to make things happen; it allows those involved to share responsibility and draw on their different skills and contacts in productive ways.

JUDY: I have felt energized by the support from the advisory committee. That's part of the beauty of CBPAR – the researcher doesn't have to know everything. We can put out questions as opposed to only answers – questions that will lead us on the path to more questions/answers and research development and recommendations leading to programmatic or service change.

The possible paths towards our desired research outcome – ultimately, equal access to healthcare for those who are marginalized by the health system – rely partially on our ability to hold various notions in tandem: subjectivities position us and our research participants unequally, and this entails particular accountabilities; but also, we are limited in our capacity to make change, often for reasons that are embedded in the very social systems we study.

Conclusions: The Limits and Challenges of Reflexivity

Emerging from our series of conversations, we reflected that the few, tentative conclusions we were able to make seem part and parcel to research processes – namely, reflection on the personal and political motivations and investments in our work is, and must be, ongoing. We did feel the conversations were beneficial in numerous ways: they reminded us of the ever-evolving nature of subjectivities and allowed us an opportunity to step back from current projects to reflect on what this looked like in our present contexts. They also helped us to see more clearly the reasons behind some of our dissonance with the broader healthcare research community by articulating that our research unit is somewhat isolated in its social justice slant; taking social equity as an entry point is quite different from simply doing cancer research *about* particular communities. Importantly, we felt that our thoughts about the concrete ruptures and disjunctures in research had the potential to challenge our 'comfortable' subject positions – to a degree. On this note, we heed Barbara Heron's cautionary analysis of the chasms between 'reflection' and 'action.' She notes:

> admitting one's privilege does not necessarily unsettle its operation. For this is a concept that has the potential to leave those who name it in a place of double comfort: the comfort of demonstrating that one is critically aware, and the comfort of *not* needing to act to undo privilege. For individuals on the other side of the privilege coin, the citing of privilege by those in dominance amounts, however inadvertently, to a reinscription of marginalization. (Heron, 2005)

For these reasons, we want to emphasize that this chapter's – and indeed this section's – reflexive focus is not an end in itself, but rather a starting point. It must be regarded not as a personal journey of self-discovery, but part of a continuous, relational exercise in applied critical analysis. What is most important is to consider how the concepts and issues discussed here shape, distort, or illuminate key elements of the research process – relationships, data gathering, analysis, knowledge production, and transformative outcomes. They recall for us the dangers in simply 'forging ahead,' for instance, with interviews and their interpretation, asking questions that are uninformed by theoretical considerations, and being complacent in our unconscious assumptions about where we come from and why we do research in the first place.

Like anyone, researchers will always make mistakes, fail to see elements of the work, miss critical nuances of power relations, and be eluded by the histories that produce us. What we *can* offer definitively at this point is that there is no way around these challenges, but the most likely route *through* is to continually unsettle the comfort zone that would frame our research as detached from the so-called 'real world' and from our own and others' lives. Moreover, vigilance about our subjectivities and investments in our work is not a therapeutic luxury, but an ethical imperative. Luckily, with the right theoretical and experiential tools, and the collaborative efforts of our research communities, we are not alone in this project.

Acknowledgments

LOWER-INCOME WOMEN WITH BREAST CANCER STUDY
Principal Investigator: Judy Gould
This project was funded by the Psychosocial and Behavioural Research Unit at the Toronto Sunnybrook Regional Cancer Centre.

WOMEN OF COLOUR LIVING WITH BREAST CANCER STUDY: BARRIERS AND BRIDGES TO SUPPORTIVE CARE
Principal Investigator: Jennifer Nelson
The Project Team: Florence Agyapong, Immigrant Women's Health Centre; Leila Springer & Winsome Johnson, The Olive Branch of Hope breast cancer support services; Sherrol Palmer-Wickham, Toronto Sunnybrook Regional Cancer Centre.

This project was funded by the Ontario Breast Cancer Community Research Initiative, which is funded by the Canadian Breast Cancer Foundation, Ontario Chapter.

NOTES

A version of this chapter was published under the title 'Hidden in the Mirror: A Reflective Conversation about Research with Marginalized Communities,'

Reflective Practice, Vol. 6, No 3, August 2005, pp. 327–39. It is reprinted with permission from Carfax Publishing, Taylor and Francis Group.

1 Cultural capital, as conceptualized by Pierre Bourdieu, refers to specific, non-economic formulations of privilege that are expressed in three states: those embodied in the individual (such as family background), those that are objectified in cultural goods (belongings, possessions), and those that are institutionalized as academic opportunities and credentials.
2 For a more thorough analysis of this issue, see Nelson, chap. 7, this volume.

REFERENCES

Abu-Lughod, L. (1991). Writing against culture. In R.G. Fox (Ed.), *Recapturing anthropology* (pp. 138–62). Santa Fe, NM: School of American Research Press.
Ahmed, S. (2000). *Strange encounters: Embodied others in post-coloniality*. London: Routledge.
Allen, D., & Cloyes, K. (2005). The language of 'experience' in nursing research. *Nursing Inquiry, 12*(2), 98–105.
Bourdieu, P. (1986). Forms of capital. In J.G. Richardson (Ed.), *Handbook of theory and research for the sociology of education* (pp. 241–55). New York: Greenwood Press.
Brah, A. (1996). *Cartographies of diaspora*. London: Routledge.
Church, K. (1995). *Forbidden narratives and critical autobiography as social science*. Amsterdam: Gordon and Breach.
Ellis, C., & Bochner, A.P. (2000). Autoethnography, personal narrative, reflexivity: Researcher as subject. In N.K. Denzin & Y.S. Lincoln (Eds.), *Handbook of qualitative research* (2nd ed.) (pp. 733–68). Thousand Oaks, CA: Sage.
Fellows, M., & Razack, S. (1998). The race to innocence: Confronting hierarchical relations among women. *Journal of Gender, Race and Justice, 1*, 335–52.
Fine, M., Weis, L., Weseen, S., & Wong, L. (2000). For whom? Qualitative research, representations, and social responsibilities. In N.K. Denzin & Y.S. Lincoln (Eds.), *Handbook of qualitative research* (2nd ed.) (pp. 107–31). Thousand Oaks, CA: Sage.
Flax, J. (1990). *Thinking fragments: Psychoanalysis, feminism, and postmodernism in the contemporary West*. Berkeley: University of California Press.
Foucault, M. (1980). Two lectures. In C. Gordon (Ed.), *Power/knowledge: Selected interviews and other writings, 1972–1977*. New York: Pantheon Books.
Foucault, M. (1982). The subject and power. *Critical Inquiry, 8*, 777–95.
Gould, J. (2004). The financial experience of lower-income women with breast

cancer: Interacting with cancer treatment and income security systems. *Canadian Woman Studies, 24*(1), 31–6.

Gunaratnam, Y. (2003). *Researching 'race' and ethnicity: Methods, knowledge and power*. London: Sage.

Hagey, R. (1997). Guest editorial: The use and abuse of participatory action research. *Chronic Diseases in Canada, 18*(1), http://www.phac-aspc.gc.ca/publicat/cdic-mcc/18-1/a_e.html

Haraway, D. (1991). *Simians, cyborgs and women: The reinvention of women*. London: Free Associated Books.

Harding, S. (1991). *Whose science, whose knowledge?* London: Open University Press.

Heron, B. (2005). Self-reflection in critical social work practice: Subjectivity and the possibilities of resistance. *Reflective Practice, 6*, 341–51.

Heron, B. (2007). *Desire for development: Whiteness, gender, and the helping imperative*. Waterloo: Wilfrid Laurier University Press.

Jeffery, D. (2002). *A terrain of struggle: Reading race in social work education* (unpublished doctoral thesis, University of Toronto).

Lather, P. (2001). Postbook: Working the ruins of feminist ethnography. *Signs, 27*(1), 199–227.

Lewis, G. (2000). *Race, gender, social welfare: Encounters in a postcolonial society*. Cambridge: Polity Press.

Malat, J. (2006). Expanding research on the racial disparity in medical treatment with ideas from sociology. *Health: An Interdisciplinary Journal for the Social Study of Health, Illness and Medicine, 10*, 303–21.

Nelson, J. (2008a). *Razing Africville: A geography of racism*. University of Toronto Press.

Nelson, J. (2008b). Lost in translation: Antiracism and the perils of knowledge. In C. Schick, J. McNinch, & L. Comeau (Eds.), *The race/culture divide in education, law and the helping professions*. University of Regina Press.

Nelson, J., & Agyapong, F. (2004). Women of colour living with breast cancer: Exploring the search for support. *Canadian Woman Studies, 24*(1), 167–72.

Smith, D.E. (1990). *The conceptual practices of power: A feminist sociology of knowledge*. University of Toronto Press

Stoetzler, M., & Yuval-Davis, N. (2002). Standpoint theory, situated knowledge and the situated imagination. *Feminist Theory, 3*, 315–33.

9 Journeying towards Authenticity: Reflections and Lessons from Our Pathways

PAMELA GRASSAU AND KARA GRIFFIN

A pathway '... marked with signposts: shifting questions and doubts, points of critical awareness, moments of celebration, and connections that demonstrate a deepening understanding of lived and transformed realities.'

–S.E. Smith, 1997, p. 11

Community-based participatory research (CBPR), a research method, process, and philosophy, has guided much of the work conducted through the Ontario Breast Cancer Community Research Initiative (OBCCRI).[1] As project coordinators who have worked with OBCCRI on two CBPR studies – Kara on the Ontario Breast Cancer Survivor Dragon Boat Study (see table 9, page 193) and Pam on the Lesbians and Breast Cancer Project (see table 7, page 122) – we propose, in this chapter, to explore the concept of 'authenticity' as an overarching core principle in the practice and process of community engagement in CBPR. 'Authenticity' has been historically aligned with participatory and liberatory theory (see McTaggart, 1997; Tandon, 1988; Wallerstein & Duran, 2003), and we suggest that it merits renewed attention for its insights as to how such theory and principles can be interwoven in the actual day to day practice of CBPR projects.

Community-based participatory research revolves centrally around the need for the community to be engaged throughout the research process: 'Community-based research in public health is a collaborative approach to research that equally involves, for example, community members, organizational representatives, and researchers in all aspects

Table 9

PSYCHOSOCIAL IMPACT OF BREAST CANCER SURVIVOR DRAGON BOATING

Why was the research completed?
Dragon boat participation by women who have been treated for breast
cancer is a growing phenomenon across Canada and the world. The
Ontario Breast Cancer Survivor Dragon Boat Study, which began in
2001, is a community-based participatory study that examined the
experiences, meaning, and psychosocial impact of dragon boating in the
lives of women with breast cancer.

What methods were used?
A mixed method, participatory research approach, guided by a community advisory group (CAG) of five survivor dragon boaters. CAG members were involved throughout all stages of the research. A group of
thirteen survivor dragon boaters also collaborated in the review and selection of standardized questionnaires for the provincial survey package.
The research involved sixty qualitative interviews with survivor dragon
boaters and a provincial survey with another four hundred dragon boaters from across Ontario.

What were the key findings?
As a survivor driven, health promotion initiative, findings indicate that
dragon boating provides a model of wellness that addresses important
intrapersonal, interpersonal, and transpersonal needs of women living
with breast cancer. In addition, dragon boating plays a meaningful and
important role in the lives of women living with breast cancer, offering
social, psychological, emotional, spiritual, and, potentially, also physical health benefits. Dragon boating also brings breast cancer survivors
out of isolation and into a community of women where they promote
individual wellness through a collective experience. The findings of our
study point to the profoundly positive impact of a comprehensive, holistic, community-based, woman-centred lifestyle for individuals who have
been diagnosed with breast cancer. Women's sense of wellness and
their quality of life is enhanced through an increased focus on the self
as they participate in a woman's team sport that incorporates emotional
expression, physical fitness, and social connectedness.

What are some implications or results of the research?
Breast cancer survivors are engaging in dragon boating to maximize
their wellness while learning to live each day of their lives to the fullest.
The lessons learned in relation to the importance of holistic programming and women's camaraderie have the potential to advance our
understanding of the promotion of women's health generally.

Further research is now being designed to test the emerging hypoth-
esis that participation in survivor boating has the potential to reduce
post-traumatic stress and cancer recurrence among women who have
been treated for breast cancer.

---

of the research process' (Israel, Schulz, Parker, & Becker, 1998, p. 177).
Tied with the need for the community to be involved in all stages is a
shared sense of a process and outcome which is 'for the purposes of
education and taking action or effecting social change' (Green et al.,
1995).

When considering community engagement in a CBPR project, an
important first step is to think about what engagement means – both
as a set of concrete tasks (for instance, building advisory groups and
having participants play an active role in the research design) and as
processes and outcomes. Engagement can also be regarded as a stage of
community-based research, where an emphasis is placed on how one
initially forms relationships with a community. 'Engaging,' here, refers
to entering a community that one may or may not be connected to, personally or professionally.

Within this chapter, we place a strong emphasis on the processes
which inform how community engagement is actualized in the community. In our experiences, community engagement is not something
that is attended to at only one phase or stage of the research; we see it
as something that needs to be attended to at all phases of a research
project, reflecting the ways in which relationships can shift and evolve
during a project.

Chapter Roadmap

We have chosen the metaphor of a 'pathway' to relay some of the key
individual and collective signposts that we encountered as we worked
towards authenticity in our two CBPR studies. Specifically we address
four key signposts that we believe are strongly interwoven when work-

ing to bring authenticity into one's CBPR practice: (1) Power and privilege, (2) Trust, (3) Voice, and (4) Reciprocity. Our overall goal is to offer students and researchers new to CBPR some concrete examples of how following CBPR theory, values, and concepts can directly benefit research practice.

The pathway represents 'engagement,' with respect to the many ways in which community members engage and re-engage throughout their projects. Along the path are 'signposts' (Smith, 1997, p. 11), which represent for us some of the core elements connected to authentic CBPR practice. Within each signpost, we offer a selection of salient questions for researchers to consider, and for one question in each section we share our own experiences, insights, and reflections from our individual projects. Our journey was not always a straightforward one, allowing us to move directly from one point to another throughout our studies; the pathway metaphor is intended to represent the process, versus the outcome, of CBPR. There have been noteworthy entry points, moments of backtracking, points for reflection, pause, and discussion.

We humbly admit that we do not have any easy answers or quick solutions to how CBPR should be practised. There are, of course, more questions than answers – but we attempt to offer some useful questions and reflections, which we hope will support and encourage the reader in a consideration of how community engagement and authenticity can be woven together in one's CBPR practice.

Defining Community

What can 'community' mean? While there are varying ways that 'community' may be defined, within many contexts, community alludes to notions of geography and context, where one envisions a group of people who live or work within a certain area. Moving the notion of communities beyond geographic parameters allows us to engage with the multiple spheres in which we live, work, and move. Communities may come together through common interests, such as political affiliations, sports, or religious/spiritual activities or practices. Communities may also reflect shared or common identities and locations, such as ethnic or cultural background, socioeconomic location, gender, or sexual orientation. Clearly, one can be a member of many different communities, and varying degrees of belonging, identification, and involvement are possible (see Godway & Finn, 1994).

Over the past decade there has been a growing CBPR literature base reinforcing the need for community-based researchers to clearly and directly articulate their own positionality, location, and power in relationship to the community and the community research (Hills & Mullett, 2000a; Israel et al., 1998; Israel et al., 2003; Lather & Smithies, 1997; McTaggart, 1997; Potvin, Cargo, McComber, Delormier, & Macaulay, 2003). Strongly supporting and reinforcing the need for this identification and reflection are core theories, principles, and values that are found across feminist, postcolonial, participatory, and action-oriented paradigms (Fonow & Cook, 1991; Reinharz, 1992). However, few examples exist that offer students and new researchers a window into thinking about how their own identities, locations, and experiences may be interconnected with the work that they engage with through community-based research. Important critical discussions need to happen to ensure that research does not become disconnected from the community.

One way of ensuring that a reflexive process is respectfully and responsibly enhancing community research is to bring reflexivity and process more centrally into the picture. As a way of speaking to this reflexive process we offer our own illustrations from each of our CBPR projects, relaying: who the communities were that were connected to each project, our own connection to each of these communities, and the context behind our roles as project co-coordinators.

The Communities

DRAGON BOAT STUDY (Kara)
The Ontario Breast Cancer Survivor Dragon Boat Study was made up of breast cancer survivors who participate in the dynamic sport of dragon boating and/or the survivor dragon boat community. This project was guided by a community advisory group of five survivor-dragon boaters and involved teams from across Ontario.

LESBIANS AND BREAST CANCER PROJECT (Pam)
The Lesbians and Breast Cancer Project was made up of lesbians and partners of lesbians directly affected by cancer, along with staff and volunteers at agencies in the lesbian/feminist and cancer communities.

Our Connection as Researchers to These Communities

Some researchers choose areas of research because of their own personal standpoint or experience. Others may find themselves involved in an unfamiliar community setting and, through community invitation or acceptance and a participatory process, develop appreciation and respect for community members' experiences. Regardless of whether one is an insider or outsider to the research community, there is power intrinsic to the researcher role, which separates the person to some extent from the community or, at the very least, redefines the CBPR relationship (Erickson, 2006; Israel et al., 1998).

It is important to identify and locate oneself as a researcher in relationship to the communities with whom one is working. This allows us to better reflect on the identities and locations that might be shared or unique across the project team.

What Is My Connection to the Lesbian Community and the Breast Cancer Community?

LESBIANS AND BREAST CANCER PROJECT (Pam)
Working in the area of breast cancer research was not new to me when I started working at OBCCRI. Breast cancer is in my family, and prior to working at OBCCRI, I had the opportunity to work with my aunt who, while living with metastatic breast cancer, was also a researcher studying the psychosocial aspects of breast cancer and genetic testing. The new layer for me in the Lesbians and Breast Cancer Project was thinking through how my own identity as 'queer' would connect to my work as the project coordinator. Listening to women's stories of heterosexism and homophobia created difficult moments of resonance and anger, while also offering incredible moments of hope and connection.

Disseminating our findings within local and cancer centre communities and using 'I/we' pronouns was and is an important aspect of my work. I have, on multiple fronts, 'come out' as I have networked and presented our findings within predominantly mainstream heterosexual environments. Each time this happens, I'm aware of the 'risk,' and yet I'm also aware that my 'coming out' happens when I have the privilege of being healthy – a stark difference from those who are coming out as they are diagnosed and/or moving through treatment/surgery or follow-up. Not having been diagnosed with breast cancer shifts my experiences radically from those of others connected to our work. I have felt humbled to have those around me share and reflect on how their diagnosis has altered their experience – for both the present and the future.

What Is My Connection to the Breast Cancer Community and
the Dragon Boat Community?

DRAGON BOAT STUDY (Kara)
When I began working at OBCCRI, while I had a strong interest in
women's health, I was new to cancer research. The experience of cancer at that time, however, was close to my heart as I had two relatives
gravely ill with cancer. One of my aunts died soon after diagnosis. My
other aunt survived an advanced cancer diagnosis. My involvement in
this study bridged the personal and the professional, and for the next
couple of years I would reflect upon the experience of cancer in wom-
en's lives more than I ever had in my life. My experience, therefore, has
been a mixed one: coloured with incredible sadness at the loss of a family member and, later, as I grew to understand the experience of survivor dragon boaters, I also learned about *living*. Many of the women I
worked with or interviewed were not focused on dying, but on living
fully and well. My aunt who died loved life, family, and community
and she recognized the importance of living joyfully. She was also an
active and health-conscious person. I can now see in her the spirit of
a dragon boater, as I do in my surviving aunt, who celebrates life and
loves to laugh and share stories.

While I've been an outsider to the personal experience of breast cancer, I have felt impacted and moved by women's stories and approaches to this disease, and an admiration for their choices. Working with
and meeting dragon boaters throughout the research process helped to
bring authenticity to our study and it also enriched my experience as a
researcher.

Our Role as Project Coordinators

We came to our CBPR projects with our own life experiences, world
views, and our formal education in graduate programs in social work
(Pam) and community psychology (Kara); also important to a research
process are the values we have been taught. Although we each worked
on different CBPR projects, we worked closely together. In addition to
sharing office space, we engaged in rich dialogue about our projects –
both challenges and triumphs at different points over the course of the
work. We were involved in all aspects of our studies; as well as the day
to day project management and consultation, we assisted with recruit-

ment, interviewing, data collection and analysis, and dissemination. We developed relationships with advisory group members and liaised with them on an ongoing basis, and we served as the link between the community/participants and the larger project team.[2]

Our Signposts

What Do We Mean by Authenticity?

Guiding values and principles have been documented throughout much of the CBPR literature (Hills & Mullett, 2000a, 2000b; Israel et al., 1998; Israel et al., 2003; McTaggart, 1997). This focus on principles and values of CBPR, rather than on concrete methods and tools, is a response to the need to understand the attitude behind CBPR (Chataway, 2001, p. 240, as cited in Kidd & Kral, 2005, p. 188). As we shared experiences from our projects, we became aware of how a broader intention to working 'authentically' was guiding much of our work. In the literature, authenticity refers to the multiple ways in which community members should be involved in all stages of the research process, and how the research process has to both begin with and belong to the community itself (McTaggart, 1997, pp. 28–9; Tandon, 1988, p. 13). This means that the research question or issues to be investigated are determined in dialogue with the community, rather than emerging only from the researcher's interests. The research plan is forged in order to explicitly respond to community goals and needs.

In research with marginalized communities, sometimes it is necessary to start simply by raising awareness in broader society about this marginalized community's needs or interests, and researchers and community members can mutually determine the best strategies for doing so given the particular project and resources. It is essential that engagement with the community be more than a token gesture or consultation about their needs, and several authors have addressed the risks of more superficial efforts (Hagey, 1997; Hatch, Moss, Saran, Presley-Cantrell, & Mallory, 1993; Moje, 2000; Reinharz, 1992; Wise, 1987). For instance, criticism has been directed towards community research projects that do not result in concrete benefits for the community involved or benefit the researchers' careers more than achieving any form of social change (Mitchell & Baker, 2005).

We attempt to take these historical lessons and critical interventions into account as we begin new projects. As such, the goal of authenticity reaffirms our responsibility as researchers to critically reflect on how our actions affect the lives of those with whom we work. This entails attending to the process of *how* we engage in our work, which is just as important as the outcomes of our projects.

In the discussion that follows, we provide some reflections and accounts related to the four elements or signposts that we signalled as central to an authentic CBPR project: (1) Power and privilege, (2) Trust, (3) Voice, and (4) Reciprocity. Within each, we introduce critical questions that we believe should be addressed by researcher/community teams before they embark on a CBPR project and throughout all of its phases. Through our responses to some of these critical questions, we share snapshots from our experiences that may have practical application and/or demonstrate lessons learned, insights, challenges, or tensions in a CBPR study.

It is important to note that these elements are not simply encountered at one point in a project. They are part of a process which also includes a focus on the project's end goals. We do not see each of these elements standing in isolation, even though each is presented as a distinct category; rather, they interweave, connect, and inform each other. Further, as noted, the elements, related questions, and applications are not exhaustive. We encourage researchers to be open to new approaches, definitions, and personal meanings.

Power and Privilege

When establishing and building researcher-participant relationships, sharing and negotiating power are central to ensuring that the process and outcomes of the project represent community voices and experiences. Indeed, power is a central thread throughout all of our relationships, particularly those within a researcher-participant/community context. As Wallerstein and Duran (2003) note, 'CBPR practice must be about asking questions and examining the power dynamics that exist when some people speak and others are silent' (pp. 38–9). It is key within a participatory process to allow for genuine involvement throughout all stages of the research. However, the sharing of power is complicated and layered and involves recognizing the privilege and responsibility of such power. For example, we needed to attend to the necessary time-consuming process of building relationships and gathering the experiences of community members while also accomplishing project goals in a timely way, and merging our own research knowledge and formal training with community knowledge and experience.

What Does It Look Like to Invite Participants' Experiences and Expertise to the Table?

DRAGON BOAT STUDY (Kara)

Our all-day research workshop is an illustration of what it can look like to invite women's perspectives to the table, to share power, and to integrate their feedback in a complex research process. For one day, we brought together a group of survivor dragon boaters, to invite their reflections on emerging qualitative findings and to seek their opinions in the creation of a survey package to be sent to hundreds of dragon boaters. On this day, we endeavoured to combine qualitative research, quantitative measures, and a participatory process. We asked them to individually review a selection of standardized questionnaires, to share their thoughts and reactions in small and large group discussions, and then to choose the questionnaires to be included in a provincial survey and to exclude those questionnaires that did not capture their experiences. Workshop participants were instrumental in a discussion of survey distribution methods and details about how to best recruit the dragon boat community to participate in the research.

We attempted to create a positive experience and an open environment that we hope fostered the sharing of power and voice as we charted some unfamiliar territory. For some it may have been the first time they had engaged in a participatory research process, and for the research team it represented a unique facilitation of a mixed-methods process, especially for qualitative researchers. Our experience shed light on how to balance research goals and perspectives with community expertise and perspectives. Our process highlighted important issues around the use of a survey method to capture knowledge and experience, as well as such questions as: Is the survey clear and relevant for those who will receive it? Does the benefit outweigh any potential harm?

Those at the workshop brought invaluable experience-based knowledge that helped to form a more complete research picture and to 'humanize' the tool or process. The community advisory group, with whom we had built a relationship over the year prior, were our compass, guiding us throughout the study and partnering with us on that day to facilitate the workshop's goals. Our experience taught us how time consuming, demanding, and complex such a process can be for the research team and, especially, for community members. But the workshop also demonstrated how a participatory process was beneficial in the creation of a study tool; through consultation, we gained important insight into what worked, what needed revision, and the best ways to reach the community and foster their participation. We also learned that the community's valuable participation cannot overshadow the physical needs that arise; it was important to offer healthy food, a comfortable environment, as well as opportunities for celebration and networking, and financial compensation for their time (Mitchell, Nielsen, Finkelstein, & Yakiwchuk, 2008; Mitchell, Chiu, & Griffin, 2004).

Other Critical Questions Related to Power and Privilege:

- How can we strive towards and work in a way that shares power?
- As researchers, are we prepared to relinquish some control and trust in a complex community process? What are the implications of relinquishing control for participants, researchers, and the project goals?
- How are you and others prepared to remain aware of your power and privilege as you work with this community?

Trust

Surprisingly, literature about CBPR rarely addresses the concept of trust. Miller (2004), in his own work with refugee communities, refers to the 'puzzling lack of discussion regarding issues of trust, access, and the relational context in the literature' (p. 217). He notes that trust 'implies the existence of an authentic interpersonal relationship' (p. 218). How, though, do we gauge whether there is trust within our relationships? In some ways, it feels more appropriate for community members than for researchers to define what trust means in a research study – what they feel needs to be in place to ensure trust between participants and researchers. Trust cannot be taught; rather, it is part of a larger process over time and, ultimately, it is critical to the overall research process. In the absence of community members' voices on trust, we share critical questions, which we feel may help to illuminate some key issues connected to trust.

Why Might Researchers Not Be Trusted?

AN EXAMPLE FROM THE LESBIANS AND BREAST CANCER PROJECT (Pam)
As I was wrapping up a research interview for the Lesbians and Breast Cancer Project, one of the women I interviewed asked, 'How do I know that ten years from now someone won't be repeating your study, as your study is gathering dust on a shelf?' Her tone, while quiet and thoughtful, pierced through me. I struggled to respond. I didn't want to make sweeping promises about how far our research would go in the world – but I also wanted her to know that the women in our project team were committed to ensuring that the research did get back to the cancer support services and health organizations that care for women with cancer. I was tentative in my response, relaying that while I couldn't predict the future, I knew that one of the ways of ensuring change is having the key organizations involved in the project team from the start. We had worked hard to ensure that our project team reflected a wide range of women, and a big part of our project meetings involved thinking about how our research results could make it back into the community in a variety of formats.

Part of her question, though, seemed to be about something bigger. She was asking whether or not she could trust us, whether or not we would ensure that her story and experience would make a difference for other lesbians with cancer. She had participated in other research, in which she felt many people had ignored her needs or negated her story – why should she trust me/us? I'm not sure I really answered this for her that day. The learning here for me is about how her question still echoes as I reflect on the research process. Perhaps this can only be addressed through our actions as researchers, by genuinely engaging with the people in our communities and by constantly asking ourselves, 'why should anyone trust us?'

Other Critical Questions Related to Trust:

- What does one need to think about or put in place when entering a community?
- How is trust best built and sustained in the research relationship? Who gives and who receives trust?
- What does ethical community entry look like within a CBPR study?

Voice

A core element of feminist theory and literature connected to CBPR is the emphasis on women giving 'voice' to their experiences (Belenky, Clinchy, Goldberger, & Tarkle, 1986; Gilligan, 1982; Lather & Smithies, 1997). This emphasis refers to the forms of knowledge that can only be gleaned by listening to others' personal experiences.

Voice, in the CBPR context, is complex and there are many ways to work within communities to capture voice, while also recognizing that fully understanding an individual or community experience does not happen in isolation or at once through a single dialogue. Community researchers strive to present authentic representations of participants' experiences and provide a glimpse into the world of those whose experiences they may not share or have not lived. However, even in CBPR, it is possible that not all participants will feel their voice or story has been fully represented, nor does community representation mean that members serve as 'representatives' of a group's experiences or views. Various theorists call for greater awareness of the complexities of representing others' experiences, particularly across important socio-political differences (Fine, Weiss, Weesen, & Wong, 2000; Gunaratnam, 2003) and for the recognition that knowledge about participants/communities is not simply observed and reported, but constructed within particular social and historical contexts (Harding, 1991).

How Do We Begin to Understand or Capture a
Participant's/Community's Voice?

AN EXAMPLE FROM THE DRAGON BOAT STUDY (Kara)

> Wild women, strong and free, missing our friends – Dragons Abreast Dragon Boat Team
>   –Memorial bench in Humber Bay Park West, Toronto

What is striking to me about the Dragon Boat study is the survivors' strong desire to bring their stories of celebration and remembrance forward in the world. Indeed, some of the women involved with or interviewed for our study were already vocal about their experiences through their passionate involvement in dragon boating. Their message existed in the public arena, as they travelled and raced throughout the world, publicly embracing the dragon boater identity and spreading the word that 'there is life after breast cancer.'

As a researcher, I felt surrounded with poignant examples of dragon boaters' voices or visibility, and had many inroads into understanding the meaning of this sport in their lives. Voice, across some traditional or community-based studies, may not be as accessible or public. An understanding of voice in the CBPR context may be shaped through a multitude of experiences and through ongoing engagement with a community.

Because of my research role and own life experience I was always outside of their experience. However, we were welcomed into the dragon boat community, especially by the community advisory group, and we were privileged to work with or meet dragon boaters at various events. Learning about dragon boating within and outside of the interview context, such as watching them race at dragon boat festivals, provided a window into the richness and layers of their experience, allowing me to appreciate it more fully. On a few occasions, I was also fortunate to travel to an interview participant's home where some shared mementoes or photos of dragon boat adventures. Their experiences, it seemed, were so much bigger than one interview could ever capture and Terry [PI] and I talked about and reflected upon their inspiring stories of transformation long after the interviews. A memorable experience for me was the opportunity to join a team one evening, and, among these athletic and strong women, I paddled for the first time on a dragon boat. I witnessed their power and community as they paddled, chanted, socialized, and laughed.

As CBPR researchers, it feels important to be mindful of both the possibilities for this type of research and of the limits of any form of research. Perhaps the lasting question we might ask ourselves, entrusted with people's stories, is whether and how we can truly know or authentically convey a person's voice and experience through our research.

Other Critical Questions Related to Voice to Consider:

- What does it mean to be in the role of narrator and 'keeper' of participants' stories? How do we address the implicit power within this role?
- How do we decide which voices are highlighted in communities that represent many different voices and locations?

- Given the profound levels of oppression that exist within a society that predominantly revolves around white, middle-class, male, heterosexual, able-bodied individuals, how do we ensure that the voices we present to the larger community do not further marginalize the people we are working with?

Reciprocity

Initially, when one refers to the term 'reciprocity,' tangible forms of compensation for community members' time and energy come to mind. 'Reciprocity implies give and take, a mutual recognition of meaning and power. It operates at two primary points in emancipatory empirical research: the junctures between researcher and researched, and between data and theory' (Lather, 1986, p. 263). Patti Lather moves the conversation beyond honoraria and thank-you gifts to consider reciprocity at deeper and more significant levels. The definition of reciprocity is ideally broadened to include a sustaining impact on the individual and a benefit to the larger community, redefining what it means to 'give back.'

What Does It Mean to Have Personal Connections to the Topic or the Community?

AN EXAMPLE FROM THE LESBIANS AND BREAST CANCER PROJECT (Pam)
When I think about reciprocity, I immediately think about how so much of my earlier social work training reinforced the importance of keeping our personal and professional lives separate. While there are clearly important reasons for thinking about how we engage with others in the community and how we move between our personal lives and our work lives, I am struck by how my life has been affected by the relationships with the women connected to our project. Perhaps it's the intimacy of breast cancer – seeing scars, holding women's hands as they hear about a recurrence; maybe it's the connections as women and as women who partner with other women – communicating about homophobic experiences, laughing about shared experiences. Regardless of the reason, I am connected in varying ways to the women who were and are part of our CBPR project.

The challenge for me is to be mindful of my own location and the power that I hold. As a paid researcher, it was important to me that the work and time of our volunteer community members were valued and that steps were taken not to abuse the commitment and dedication of the community members. When women connected to our study were asked to take part in the dissemination of our findings across the province, a primary component was to try to ensure that they could be paid adequately for their time. After planning multiple back-to-back presentations to meet the needs of one of the organizations we were working with, it was clear that we had over-taxed the community members who were part of our dissemination presentation. The take-away message for us was that we needed to prioritize the health and well-being of the women from our communities as we disseminated our findings.

Other Critical Questions Related to Reciprocity:

- How does the concept of reciprocity in community research differ from that in traditional research?
- How does reciprocity change how relationships are built? How can research truly contribute to the communities with whom we work?
- Are there explicit dialogues with the community, research team, or funder about specific expectations for the project? What are the limits of the research?
- Is one being sensitive to the needs of community members and mindful of the amount of time/energy that is being asked of them?

Thus far, we have offered our own learning related to what we feel are four essential elements of authentic community engagement: (1) Power and privilege, (2) Trust, (3) Voice, and (4) Reciprocity. Our hope is that these reflections and critical questions will lead to even more questions for readers and other researchers. Ultimately, we hope that our reflections will encourage more researchers to write about their own learning, offering their own questions, insights, and challenges for all engaged in CBPR.

Further Considerations for CBPR

At the beginning of any journey, we typically map out a plan and put in place some basic components – those things to help us navigate the geography while factoring in time, travel, basic self-care needs, perhaps even contingencies – all to facilitate a healthy, positive, and meaningful experience. A community research project is no exception. Throughout this chapter, we have suggested that, in addition to mapping out a practical research timeline, research questions, and project deliverables, we begin to think more broadly and foster dialogues that attend to critical questions related to the community and the team.

It feels appropriate to end this chapter where it began, and so we return to the metaphor of a pathway and to our goal of working towards authentic engagement as an overarching principle of CBPR. Time has a way of offering important space to reflect on what worked well, as well as what one would do differently as one moves on to other projects. Based on our experiences and reflections, we part with some final considerations that we feel may be absent or inadequately addressed within CBPR literature and discussions.

Time, Time, Time

CBPR is a complex and intensive endeavour, requiring much time, flexibility, and dedication on the part of the research team. It is critical to build in extra time up-front for relationship-building and engagement with a community, even if this community is familiar. One of the greatest challenges to doing community-based research, especially that with an 'action' agenda, is outlining a realistic plan that can be accomplished within the time and financial limits of the grant – a plan that will also be useful to the research team and allow them to fulfil grant goals while addressing and furthering a community agenda.

Questions Related to Time:

- Is there extra time built into the CBPR project in case certain activities take longer than anticipated?
- As a project team, what specifically – activities, goals, plans, processes – is the team willing to be flexible about, and what needs to stick to a firm timeline?
- How does the project fit within a longer-term community plan? Which goals connect to the CBPR project, directly or in the near future, and which are longer term and require new initiatives to see them realized?

Importance of Remembrance and Celebration

In our experiences with community-based cancer research, it was important to acknowledge how central sorrow, loss, and grief are to women's lives. During the Lesbians and Breast Cancer Project, we incorporated a memorial service into one of our project team meetings to acknowledge and honour the death of one of our founding project team members. Within the Dragon Boat Study, we observed a carnation ceremony at the end of a dragon boat race, where women throw carnations into the water to remember those who have died.

Opportunities for project team and community celebrations, such as listening to dragon boat race stories, celebrating positive health reports, and completing specific phases of the research, were key to enriching our participatory research projects.

Questions Related to Remembrance and Celebration:

- How would the community define and integrate elements of significance and celebration into the process/tasks of the CBPR project?
- How can genuine celebration be integrated throughout the CBPR project?

Disengagement

While much literature exists on the process of community engagement in participatory projects, there is very little dialogue about what it means to exit or disengage at the end of a study (Northway, 2000). As project coordinators, we feel the need for more explicit discussion of the process and impact of leaving or ending a project. While we support the practice of building longer-term relationships within communities, which extend beyond grant/funding deadlines, it is unrealistic not to talk about how relationships will shift as projects come to a close or as contract staff leave. Even when CBPR projects continue to grow and evolve after the initial research wraps up, the end of the initial project phase is an important time at which to both acknowledge the work done and to 'mark' a transition in the group process.

Questions Related to Disengagement:

- How can all phases of the CBPR project, from beginning to end, be integrated into discussions from the beginning?
- Who is willing to carry the work forward over the long term?
- How do we ensure that community members who may be marginalized and isolated remain supported as CBPR projects shift and change?

Summary

This chapter has adopted the metaphor of a pathway, focusing largely on our process of working towards authenticity in community engagement, offering 'signposts,' critical questions, and excerpts from our research journeys. By moving through our experiences, we have come to a place in our community research practices where, alongside the many lessons learned, ongoing reflections and questions linger.

On some level, we wish we could provide comprehensive 'how-to' steps to the reader and the new community researcher, which we feel would have benefited us in graduate school. The reality is that, while there are important resources available that address CBPR,[3] there is no such guide for community research, no such exhaustive list that is transferable across diverse communities and projects. The emergent and responsive nature of community research is its strength, and it also makes for challenging work as one begins to engage with CBPR.

Every project and every community is different, with its own needs, agendas, and cultures. Researchers must take the time to be immersed in a community/culture and to make project decisions based in, and guided by, the community. What we have offered are some examples, approaches, and considerations rooted in personal experiences. We hope, as we strive to engage authentically in CBPR, that our endeavours will continue to lead us on new and instructive pathways.

Acknowledgments

LESBIANS AND BREAST CANCER: A PARTICIPATORY RESEARCH PROJECT
The Project Team: Maureen Aslin, Jennifer Alexander, Lisa Barnoff, Pauline Bradbrook, Michèle Clarke, Teri Henderson, Pam Grassau, Patti McGillicuddy, Fran Odette, Samantha Sarra, Chris Sinding, Anna Travers, Danielle Vandezande
Women who participated in the study: Lillian, Mary Lou, Marcia, Kate, Sarah, Rosalie, Maureen, Paula, Paddy, Pauline, Jessica, Paula K., Glenda, Constance, Sherry, Liz, Teagan, Gerrie, Marie, Jacquie, Jann, Lou, Bonnie, Theresa, Laura, Anette
Partner Agencies: The 519 Church Street Community Centre, DAWN Ontario: DisAbled Women's Network Ontario, The Coalition for Lesbian & Gay Rights in Ontario, Gilda's Club, The Metropolitan Community Church of Toronto, The Ontario Breast Cancer Community Research

Initiative, The Rainbow Health Network, Sherbourne Health Centre, Sunnybrook & Women's College Health Sciences Centre – Social Work & Professional Advisory Committee, Willow Breast Cancer Support & Resource Services

This project was funded by the Canadian Breast Cancer Foundation, Ontario Chapter.

PSYCHOSOCIAL IMPACT OF BREAST CANCER SURVIVOR DRAGON
BOATING STUDY
Principal Investigator: Terry Mitchell
Project Team: Ross Gray, Marg Fitch, Edmee Franseen, Kara Griffin
Advisory Committee: Franci Finkelstein, Dragons Abreast, Toronto; Bonnie Marshall, Warriors of Hope, North Bay; Eleanor Nielsen, Dragons Abreast, Toronto; Doris Rossi, Dragons of Hope, Thunder Bay; Donnas Stuart, Dragons of Hope, Thunder Bay

This project was funded by the Canadian Breast Cancer Foundation, Ontario Chapter.

NOTES

1 The OBCCRI was created in 2001 to explore, understand, and improve women's psychosocial experience of breast cancer. This unit is one of the first major Canadian research initiatives to focus on the daily lives of women with breast cancer from the perspectives of these women. Our researchers are especially committed to learning about the experiences of, and attempting to change iatrogenic health system processes for, women from marginalized groups who have also been diagnosed with breast cancer.
2 It would be impossible for us to talk about our role as project coordinators without also situating ourselves in relationship to the principal investigators of each of our CBPR projects: Dr. Terry Mitchell (Dragon Boat Study) and Dr. Christina Sinding (Lesbians and Breast Cancer Project). Both brought a strong sense of authenticity, integrity, and commitment to the work, ensuring that the community values reflected within our projects were also reflected in their relationships with each of us as coordinators. Our ability to write this chapter comes as a result of their continued commitment and integrity towards CBPR values and the creation of a research culture that provided mentoring, wisdom, and support in finding our own voices.
3 See reference list.

REFERENCES

Belenky, M.F., Clinchy, B.M., Goldberger, N.R., & Tarkle, J.M. (1986). *Women's ways of knowing: The development of self, voice, and mind.* New York: Basic Books.

Chataway, C.J. (2001). Negotiating the observer-observed relationship: Participatory action research. In D.L. Tolman & M. Brydon-Miller (Eds.), *From subjects to subjectivities: A handbook of interpretive and participatory methods* (pp. 239–55). New York University Press.

Erickson, F. (2006). Studying side by side: Collaborative action ethnography in educational research. In G. Spindler & L. Hammond (Eds.), *Innovations in educational ethnography: Theory, methods, and results* (pp. 235–57). Mahwah, NJ: Lawrence Erlbaum.

Fine, M., Weis, L., Weseen, S., & Wong, L. (2000). For whom? Qualitative research, representations, and social responsibilities. In N.K. Denzin & Y.S. Lincoln (Eds.), *Handbook of Qualitative Research* (2nd ed.) (pp. 107–31). Thousand Oaks, CA: Sage.

Fonow, M.M., & Cook, J.A. (Eds.). (1991). *Beyond methodology: Feminist scholarship as lived research.* Bloomington: Indiana University.

Gilligan, C. (1982). *In a different voice: Psychological theory and women's development.* Cambridge, MA: Harvard University Press.

Godway, E.M., & Finn, G. (Eds.). (1994). *Who is this 'we'? Absence of community.* Montreal, QC: Black Rose Books.

Green, L.W., George, A., Daniel, M., Frankish, C.J., Herbert, C.P., Bowie, W.R., et al. (1995). *Study of participatory research in health promotion: Review and recommendations for the development of participatory research in health promotion in Canada.* Ottawa, ON: Royal Society of Canada.

Gunaratnam, Y. (2003). *Researching 'race' and ethnicity: Methods, knowledge and power.* London: Sage.

Hagey, R. (1997). Guest editorial: The use and abuse of participatory action research. *Chronic Diseases in Canada, 18*(1). Retrieved from http://www.phac-aspc.gc.ca/publicat/cdic-mcc/18-1/a_e.html

Harding, S. (1991). *Whose science, whose knowledge? Thinking from women's lives.* Ithaca: Cornell University Press.

Hatch, J., Moss, N., Saran, A., Presley-Cantrell, L., & Mallory, C. (1993). Community research: Partnership in black communities. *American Journal of Preventive Medicine, 9,* 27–31.

Hills, M., & Mullett, J. (2000a). *Community-based research: Collaborative action for health and social change.* Victoria, BC: Community Health Promotion Coalition, University of Victoria.

Hills, M., & Mullett, J. (2000b, May 15–17). *Community-based research: Creating evidence-based practice for health and social change.* Paper presented at the Qualitative Evidence-based Practice Conference, Coventry University.

Israel, B.A., Schulz, A.J., Parker, E.A., & Becker, A.B. (1998). Review of community-based research: Assessing partnership approaches to improve public health. *Annual Review of Public Health, 19,* 173–202.

Israel, B.A., Schulz, A.J., Parker, E.A., Becker, A.B., Allen III, A.J., & Guzman, J.R. (2003). Critical issues in developing and following community based participatory research principles. In M. Minkler & N. Wallerstein (Eds.), *Community-based participatory research for health* (pp. 53–79). San Francisco, CA: Jossey-Bass.

Kidd, S.A., & Kral, M.J. (2005). Practicing participatory action research. *Journal of Counseling Psychology, 52*(2), 187–95.

Lather, P. (1986). Research as praxis. *Harvard Educational Review, 56*(3), 257–77.

Lather, P.A., & Smithies, C. (1997). *Troubling the angels: Women living with HIV/AIDS.* Colorado: Westview Press.

McTaggart, R. (1997). Guiding principles for participatory action research. In R. McTaggart (Ed.), *Participatory action research: International contexts and consequences* (pp. 25–43). State University of New York Press.

Miller, K.E. (2004). Beyond the frontstage: Trust, access, and the relational context in research with refugee communities. *American Journal of Community Psychology, 33*(3/4), 217–28.

Mitchell, T., & Baker, E. (2005). Culturally acceptable research community-building versus career-building research: The challenges, risks, and responsibilities of conducting research with Aboriginal and Native American communities. *Journal of Cancer Education, 20* (Suppl.), 41–6.

Mitchell, T., Chiu, C., & Griffin, K. (2004). Ontario breast cancer survivor dragon boat study: The story of our participatory and mixed methods process. Poster presentation at the 2nd Quebec–Ontario Conference in Community Psychology. Université Laval, Quebec.

Mitchell, T., Nielsen, E., Finkelstein, F., & Yakiwchuk, C. (2008). Lessons learned about women's health and wellness from survivor dragon boaters. In D. Driedger & M. Owen (Eds.), *Dissonant disabilities: Women with chronic illness theorize their lives.* Toronto: Canadian Scholars' Press.

Moje, E.B. (2000). Changing our minds, changing our bodies: Power as embodied in research relations. *International Journal of Qualitative Studies in Education, 13*(1), 25–42.

Northway, R. (2000). Ending participatory research? *Journal of Learning Disabilities, 4*(1), 27–36.

Potvin, L., Cargo, M., McComber, A., Delormier, T., & Macaulay, A. (2003).

Implementing participatory intervention and research in communities: Lessons from the Kahnawake Schools Diabetes Prevention Project in Canada. *Social Science & Medicine, 56,* 1295–306.

Reinharz, S. (1992). *Feminist methods in social research.* Oxford: Oxford University Press.

Smith, S.E. (1997). Introduction: Participatory action-research within the global context. In S.E. Smith, D.G. Willms, & N.A. Johnson (Eds.), *Nurtured by knowledge: Learning to do participatory action-research* (pp. 1–12). New York: The Apex Press.

Tandon, R. (1988). Social transformation and participatory research. *Convergence, 21*(2/3), 5–14.

Wallerstein, N., & Duran, B. (2003). The conceptual, historical, and practice roots of community based participatory research and related participatory traditions. In M. Minkler & N. Wallerstein (Eds.), *Communty-based participatory research for health* (pp. 27–52). San Francisco, CA: Jossey-Bass.

Wise, S. (1987). A framework for discussing ethical issues in feminist research: A review of the literature. *Studies in Sexual Politics, 19,* 47–88.

10 Survivor, Activist, Advocate: Reflecting on Advisory Committee Roles

PATTI MCGILLICUDDY, FALIA DAMIANAKIS,
ANN WRAY HAMPSON, AND JUDY GOULD

Participatory action research (PAR) is a form of research that aims to place the 'research capabilities in the hands of the ... disenfranchised people so that they can transform their lives for themselves' (Hagey, 1997, p. 1). The fundamental values associated with accomplishing this type of research include that the process is participatory, a collaboration between community members and researchers; a mutual learning experience, an opportunity to build capacity and increase self-determination; and an opportunity to strike a balance between research and action (Minkler, 2004). Embedded within this methodology is the principle that the stakeholder or involved community member has valued knowledge about the issue under study and about their own and their constituents' needs (Minkler). PAR projects can include the participation of an advisory committee composed of stakeholders who might participate in the research project by shaping the research question/process, helping with recruitment, discussing the findings, determining what is most meaningful or valid in the data, disseminating the findings, and helping to translate the findings into changed practice (Minkler; Porter, Parsons, & Robertson, 2006).

This chapter is the synthesis of a discussion among three women (the first three authors) working on research advisory committees as cancer survivors and community members with a psychosocial breast cancer research unit – the Ontario Breast Cancer Community Research Initiative (OBCCRI).[1] OBCCRI is supported by an advisory committee, in which Patti and Falia have participated since 2001. This advisory committee includes members from community agencies, healthcare professionals, researchers, and cancer care advocates, as well as representatives from its funder – the Canadian Breast Cancer Foundation,

Ontario Chapter (CBCF, ON). Falia and Patti were associated with this research unit because the creators of the unit actively sought the participation of cancer survivors who also held a stated interest and professional skills in cancer care.

The advisory committee acts as a consulting body, offering advice and direction about OBCCRI research and its dissemination. Members offer important contacts from their various networks, which have often led to research partnerships or assisted with participant recruiting. At committee meetings, members are apprised of research developments, presented with particular questions, and asked to provide feedback as well as updates from their own professional and volunteer sectors. This consultation with the advisory committee helps to ensure that the research remains relevant and accountable to the participant communities.

In addition, specific research advisory committees support many of the individual OBCCRI research studies. In different capacities, the authors have also worked with these studies: Patti has been part of the Lesbians and Cancer advisory committee (see table 7, page 122), Ann participated on the Older Women with Breast Cancer advisory committee (see table 5, page 78), and Falia participated in the dissemination of the research-based drama, *Ladies in Waiting? Life after Breast Cancer*[2] (see table 11, page 242).

To prepare for this chapter we wanted to think about what it has been like to work in an advisory role with a psychosocial research unit that focuses on survivors' experiences of cancer and cancer care. We asked one of the initiative's researchers and the last author of this chapter, Judy, to facilitate our discussion, which was audio-taped and then transcribed. Over the course of the discussion, we endeavoured to address the following overarching questions:

- Why did we become involved as advisory members in the research unit or its projects?
- What has our experience been like on advisory committees?
- What is the context for this work and our role in it?
- What impact does being a survivor have on what we bring to the research advisory process?
- How and why is it important for survivors to be involved in participatory research?
- What kinds of changes have we seen in the cancer community over time?

• What tips would we provide to those thinking about involving survivors on research advisory committees?

In what follows, we have focused on some questions that guided our
discussion within the parameters of the overarching issues. We have
distilled the conversation into four main themes. We first discuss our
multiple identities and roles as members of advisory groups who are
also cancer survivors, and who, as well, have particular professional
skills and interests in the cancer community. Here, we address how and
why we became involved in this work and what we see as its major con-
tributions. Second, we talk about shifts we have noticed in the cancer
'landscape' since our diagnoses and/or since we have become involved
in research and community contexts as activists. This discussion encompasses changes – or sometimes the lack thereof – in patient information,
patient-centred decision-making, societal attitudes, and medical attitudes, all of which affect the process and content of the research.

In the third section, we reflect on our unique position as cancer survivors involved in research *about* other survivors, and the embedded
tensions around subjectivity and objectivity, connection and distance
in this process. We conclude our conversation by thinking about what
researchers and survivor advisory members need to consider when
planning to work together – for instance, what are the criteria for an
advisory member's involvement, what is it important to know about
the various voices around the table, and what are some cautions to keep
in mind, to ensure that everyone is able to contribute.

We present our discussion through first person excerpts, and then
summarize and reflect on our musings in a common voice, sometimes
at the beginning and at the end of each of the four sections.

Introductions: Multiple Identities, Roles, Perspectives, and Visions

Q: Why did you become involved with this research group?

PATTI: As a survivor of cancer, who also works in the healthcare system, I had a lot of frustration with how things worked for myself
and how things worked for the women I saw going through the
cancer system. I felt like I could make a contribution to some discussions about those two worlds – the world of healthcare and the
world of women dealing with cancer diagnoses. When I participated specifically as an advisory member with the Lesbians and Breast

Cancer Project there was also a chance to reflect on my own experience as a lesbian with cancer. I found that being an advisory member gave me the opportunity to feel more integrated in my work, to bring together both my skills and my experience as a cancer survivor, and that doesn't usually happen ...

ANN: I became involved with the Older Women and Cancer Project as an interviewer and advisory member because I found it interesting – it was like having similar experiences at two levels, one having had cancer and the other being an age-mate to the people who were the research participants. It wasn't new material because most of what I do is around working with people dealing with change and loss ... but it was exciting; I mean there was a reward in doing it ... I examined my own beliefs a lot in the process of doing it. I also felt it was important to be part of a process to effect additional change that can't be made at the individual level.

FALIA: My agreement to participate on the OBCCRI advisory committee evolved out of an extension of the work I was already doing. I had been involved in the development and the implementation of Willow Breast Cancer Support Services and I remember when the Psychosocial Behavioural Research Unit had the opportunity to develop a research unit focused on the lived experience of marginalized women the focus of that new unit mirrored what was happening at a peer support level – in community organizations like Willow. I saw that there was a real need and I very much wanted to be involved and engaged in that process. I look at it in the context of my survivorship and as an activist ... I wanted to have some kind of impact and I realized that providing support and information includes an 'activist' component. It was vital to me to be involved in creating quantitative and qualitative information, and then make an impact on how professionals can get that information out to the broader community.

Q: Would you say that advisory committees that include survivors can make a difference in getting the research out into the broader cancer community – and if so, how? What does the role look like to you?

FALIA: That makes me think of the *Ladies in Waiting? Life after Breast Cancer* research-based theatre project ... it occurred at a time where we had begun to recognize the struggles of diagnosis, treatment, and recovery, but we hadn't had exposure around the longer-term survivorship issue. So bringing the survivorship issues out into the community in a play format and having a discourse around these issues was, for me as an advocate, very powerful – seeing the impact of that research disseminated in an accessible way.

ANN: I think the topics that are being looked at by the research unit are aspects of experience about which the larger community is incurious ... previously women's experiences had often been discounted, which accounts for the lack of resources to address them.

PATTI: At the beginning, OBCCRI asked its advisory committee to be involved in the development of the strategic plan. I think the involvement of survivors in this process allowed for that visibility to remain in some kind of way, to help counteract that 'discounting' that you talk about, Ann ...

ANN: It's no longer just academic.

PATTI: Yes, if it remains simply academic, the nature of the research will change, it won't be embedded in people's experience, in women's experience, it will end up ...

ANN: ... In dusty file cabinets.

PATTI: Exactly ... And I think another piece for me becomes 'who do I represent on these advisory committees?' For example, am I doing a good job of that? Am I representing survivors, am I representing myself, am I representing myself at ten o'clock in the morning that day in terms of how I'm feeling? Do I have a responsibility to represent others, to bring those other voices to the table? And often I feel that I do, but I also recognize that it's a different kind of advocacy to bring those questions forward, to work towards more inclusion, while keeping in mind that you cannot champion the issues of all women with cancer.

FALIA: It's true. It's almost like you have to go out into the community as an 'ambassador' for the research unit, even though you may be employed by another service or you have another advocacy role as well.

ANN: ... and there's also representing the research itself – the responsibility that comes with that task.

PATTI: Yes, and it has been important to think about what that role looks like. Sometimes, the organizational culture and the way committees evolve can have a particular influence on our participation. For example, over time in the OBCCRI advisory meetings, there was a tendency for the researchers to update or report to the committee, rather than using us to brainstorm, consult and strategize as we had at the beginning. We were able to point out this trend and the meeting content broadened to include consultation as well as research updates. This has had important benefits on both sides, and I think it gives us a deeper appreciation for the research process, making us better able to represent the work.

COMMON VOICE
The perspective we bring to our 'advising' includes the eye of the survivor, the reflections based on similar experiences and the seasoned awareness of challenges and inequities in cancer diagnosis, treatment, and the ongoing tasks of living. We share a counselling and social services orientation and an activist's sensitivity to shared needs.

We come to the meetings and listen and contribute in order to avoid the 'dusty filing cabinet syndrome,' to respect the experiences of the women who have taken part in the studies, and to appreciate the researchers' academic diligence. We want to represent the research and move the results to improve practices, address social inequities, and build responsive systems for women and their families. We have acquired a sense of responsibility for the research directions and outcomes – which we perhaps did not expect to acquire, but there it is.

Still, we are aware that we do not – nor could we – represent the full spectrum of women who deal with their own journeys through the cancer system realizing that the characteristics associated with 'participation are inherently unstable, requiring constant negotiation of ideas, values, identities and interests among all who participate' (Yoshihama & Carr, 2002, p. 85), a point we will return to in the discussion of the third theme. We work towards an inclusion of all women in the community and thus become not only interested in consulting regarding this research but in championing the research itself.

Stepping Back: Shifts in Survivor Advocacy over Time

It was also important for us to speak about our journeys as survivors, facilitators, and activists in the context of cancer care and the evolution of social issues over time. Research is propelled and circumscribed by the historical context. For example, in the health realm, research into the lived experience of an illness from the perspective of a survivor as a participant was unheard of prior to the 1990s (Canadian Advisory Council on the Status of Women, 1995). Stakeholder involvement in breast cancer research and lived experience research about breast cancer are relatively new phenomena. The historical context is relevant as it provides a sense of how far citizen-participation as a process in the realm of health has come since the 1990s.

In Canada, citizens have participated to a great extent in the formal healthcare system particularly in the breast cancer movement (Sinding & Cohen, 1996). Bolstered by the gains achieved in the women's movement to understand how this disease was tainted by gender inequality (Brown & Zavestoski, 2004), Canadian women with breast cancer essentially lobbied the federal government to create a multi-million-dollar funding pocket for research. This organization also co-sponsored the National Forum on Breast Cancer in 1993 at which survivors, researchers, and decision-makers tackled the prioritizing of issues in prevention and screening, treatment and care, research and support, and advocacy (Sinding & Cohen).

Q: What sorts of shifts have you noticed in the cancer community over the last number of years?

PATTI: Twenty-five years ago, the AIDS and women's movements opened the door for more discussion and more challenges to the healthcare system. There was an attempt to see that people have lives outside of that system and the right to a relationship with that system – a relationship that addresses some of our psycho-social needs, as well as our needs around the management, quote unquote, of the disease process. We're still not there yet in terms of that kind of relationship that is more open. I think 'patient-focused care' is more about leaving things to the patient that the health professionals don't care about. I think from working inside the healthcare system, I'm still very sceptical about what's changed and what hasn't changed, but I think what has happened is that a lot of healthcare has shifted out of the hospital and into the community and onto the Internet.

FALIA: I am hopeful that patients have made some progress in terms of encouraging health professionals to participate in community-driven initiatives. In the mid-1990s physicians didn't like that survivor-driven organizations were creating patient information brochures – they

didn't want to do medical presentations around an issue to a lay population, and they weren't going to be collaborators or partners in a
survivor-driven organization. Is there ever a shift now! You're seeing
physicians, oncologists, and researchers on boards of directors and on
advisory committees for community-based cancer support agencies,
doing presentations to lay audiences. This is the exciting side.

ANN: I am going to credit the survivor movement for that shift. But it's
not about attacking the health professionals. Experience has made
us more aware of the hardships and struggles that physicians face
in providing service, so we want to make sure that we give voice
to both sides – both patients and physicians have difficulties. The
other societal shift is that more women are involved in more positions and responsibilities than they used to be. And these women
are prepared to speak up.

COMMON VOICE

It is important to understand our place in time to continually assess
our own power and limitations as survivors, as activists, as facilitators,
and as women. We benefit from awareness of the literature and the rich
experience of those who work as survivors or representatives in health
and social movements such as those movements that are focused on
improving access to health services (universal insurance reform), illuminating the experience of disease or disability (breast cancer movement, AIDS activism), or drawing attention to and activism against
health inequality/inequity (women's health movements, gay and lesbian health movement) within which traditional structures of authority
(science, medicine) are challenged (Brown & Zavestoski, 2004). Lessons
from knowledge of or participation in these other movements help us
to contextualize the experience of the individual in the process of de-
mocratizing knowledge.

We understand that we are part of larger political and social movements, which inform cancer care and influence its impact, so the ability
to effect improvements in care is not only about the effectiveness of
the research or strategy, but also depends on the social climate of the
time. We have seen important shifts over the last two decades with regard to the patient's role in cancer care and the number of services and
support available to middle- to upper-class cancer survivors (Klawiter,
2004). In some ways, the medical profession has opened to the possibility of greater patient participation in their own health care. Yet, we
have remaining concerns as to the role of community groups and other

information sources, such as the Internet. Patients are empowered to understand more, to make decisions and act in their own interests, but does this simply displace the responsibilities of the medical system onto community and informal networks? We are, alternately, encouraged and concerned about the state of progress around cancer information, patient access, decision-making, and healthcare provider involvement in community awareness and education.

The historical shifts to focus on patient-centred care have also had an impact in shaping the process and format of patient-centred research. Following the seminal meeting in 1993, the National Forum on Breast Cancer, the federal government funded the Canadian Breast Cancer Research Initiative (CBCRI) wherein this research funder agreed to:

> address the priorities brought forward by women ... The participation of lay women and breast cancer survivors on the management committee is a vital feature of the CBCRI that helps to ensure that the priorities and concerns of patients and their families are kept at the forefront while the integrity of rigorous scientific investigation is maintained. (Hagen & Whylie, 1998)

The construction of this funding body has inevitably resulted in an increase in survivor participation in breast cancer research in Canada.

Shared Identity on the 'Moving Sidewalk': The Objective/Subjective Dance

Q: What is it like to be participating in research about cancer patients and survivors when you are survivors yourselves?

ANN: There are fuzzy edges to this work. When I interviewed women who were my age-mates and who had also had cancer, I felt like we were riding an irreversible moving sidewalk – we weren't always in the same 'place'; our points of connection were always shifting. So at some points during the interview I felt comfortable and at other points I felt less comfortable. Interviewing folks who have had similar experiences is like a dance between the objective and subjective, because we're really aiming towards objective information, but we're using our subjective selves to do it.

FALIA: So this goes back to the multiple roles that we have to juggle. One informs the other ...

PATTI: Yes, because we do share the identity of 'survivor' so being on that moving sidewalk may not be that comfortable for us.

ANN: It is often like going back into the trenches.

PATTI: Yeah it is. It is …

FALIA: And then again, ten years post-diagnosis, I do not feel as though I am re-entering the trenches. I have a sense of feeling normal – no longer a cancer survivor. I can hear all about the feelings in the trenches but I don't feel like I'm re-entering all that vulnerability which I had lived with for years. But then I question, 'Am I a good representative for the cancer survivor?'

ANN: I feel I cannot escape that vulnerability because of what I might have handed down to my children. I think that is common among people who are parents, particularly if it's something that tends to run in families … Even if it feels like history for me, it's not history for my children.

PATTI: It's sort of living with the recognition that we are all fragile, as human beings.

ANN: Absolutely, and I think it's just that you've got some concrete form for that fragility to be at the front of your brain.

FALIA: Sometimes it feels like it's at the front, and sometimes I feel more removed from the immediacy of the emotional response of what it's like to be diagnosed. It's that feeling of a shifting identity again. I see my involvement in the cancer community less as a survivor now, and more in a professional role applying the same skills that I would have if I were working in an area other than cancer. Sometimes I'm more objective about certain things than I used to be, and that's when I question if I can be a representative, to carry the passion and the thrust of the breast cancer movement, the passion that happens in the trenches.

PATTI: Perhaps there is room for everyone.

ANN: Yes … We really have a spectrum of connections. I think that people who are newly diagnosed benefit greatly from meeting others who are newly diagnosed – from being able to speak in the particular language of those early days – and I also think that being able to meet with people who are at a different stage offers another connection.

COMMON VOICE

The dance between the objective and the subjective is something we can all relate to in this process. Perhaps it is not unlike the research process itself with all its inherent challenges. We see ourselves and others in the

work completed – or, at times, we do not. We sometimes see unanticipated connections or differences, and we use the surprises to inform the
next steps in our relationships and our work. We try to get the word out
so there is more help, support, information, and knowledge for women
surviving cancer. This means, ultimately, more for *us* too.

Being both the subject and object of a research enterprise is sometimes daunting, sometimes integrative, sometimes surprising, and
sometimes tiring. The analogy of the moving sidewalk, drawn initially
by Ann in reference to the Older Women study, rings true for many of
our experiences as survivors researching survivors. Our points of connection with others – as, for example, women who have had cancer, as
someone in the same age group, or as a lesbian – might seem relatively
straightforward, but the common 'sidewalks' on which we move with
other women keep shifting as we take up different roles in our advisory work. At one point we might share a similar pathway; at another
point we might be in the position of interviewer; at yet another time, we
might be in the position of 'outsiders,' observing others' experiences in
what is presumed to be an objective light. We must constantly negotiate
the complexities both of identity itself and of how identity shifts over
time with new and familiar roles.

When engaging in qualitative research the research team is charged
with respectfully retelling the story of the participant – a task that requires deep attention and engagement with the research process and
content (Jones, 2002). The pursuit of getting the story 'right' is complicated at the best of times with our own stories. Michelle Fine (1994)
refers to this experience as 'working the hyphen' of self-other in which
the hyphen 'both separates and merges personal identities with our in-
ventions of Others' (p. 70).

This is further complicated for us survivor-researchers who have had
the experience as patient/survivors of having our stories discounted
or objectified, parsed, scrutinized. As advisory members, survivors are
tied to cancer in an essential way making us both privy and more vulnerable to a deeper understanding of the cancer story while recognizing that we have cancer experiences that are dissimilar to others (Porter
et al., 2006, also consider this finding).

Working the hyphen then requires perhaps even more diligence or
reflection from those survivor-researchers (as compared to outsider-
researchers) whose personal experiences move, collide, are shaped and
reshaped by our (dis)connection with research participants during the
research process (Gunaratnam, 2003).

Concluding Tips for the Inclusion of Survivors as Research Advisory Group Members

We had hoped, through this conversation, to provide some guidance from our own experiences for researchers about forming advisory committees and how best to facilitate their function in research projects. But what we had envisioned as a list of handy tips, 'dos and don'ts', or a checklist of sorts, took a few different turns. We spoke about the entry points for participation, the politics of choice, and the defined roles for advisors and advisees in research organizations with a participatory research approach.

Q: What advice would you give researchers who would like to involve cancer survivors in projects or on advisory committees? Are there particular rules of engagement or guidelines for who should participate and how?

FALIA: This relates to the point that you, Patti, were raising about giving women tips who want to enter this work as advisory group members. Is it being a cancer survivor that's important or is it the other set of skills that we bring in that precedes our cancer?

PATTI: And if, previous to the cancer experience, we had been perhaps a physical education teacher, or we had worked in construction, or done work at home we might have the same passion for change but we might have expressed it in a different way. We might or might not have joined this research unit – we might have started a dragon boat team.

FALIA: Right ... and so the kinds of tips we might give a woman who was in a discipline unrelated to what the three of us have in common (social services, counselling) may look quite different.

PATTI: And I think that maybe, then, when you're looking at having advisors on research projects, there's an advantage probably to both – people who have that affinity for this kind of research that predates their cancer diagnosis and then also people who bring a fresh perspective – we need to look for diversity, difference, unique energies and views.

Q: What groundwork, would you suggest, can be done to help ensure that survivor committee members have a good experience?

FALIA: Well, the selection process and how you advise women about becoming involved as committee members might depend on many variables. I think it's fair to ask 'What about your skills? What are you bringing in?' – it is not just because they've had the cancer experience that they should participate, because at times, the emotional impact can be overwhelming.

ANN: We need to have parameters in selecting people, looking at emotional preparedness as well as history and skills. There are many pieces to this.

PATTI: It points to the need for providing supports to survivor-advisory members. Sometimes in research with physically or socially vulnerable women you are looking for advisory members who have had similar experiences. So I guess the question then becomes how do you support these women to participate on advisory committees? I think about the Lesbians and Cancer Project in particular, in which the degree of support and facilitation that participants required was quite profound. They needed money for childcare, transportation, attendants, and multiple meeting breaks for those who were tired due to treatment and medication. These issues will come to the fore when people come to participate as advisory members.

FALIA: Especially if you want marginalized groups represented on advisory committees – you have to make sure that you level the playing field by offering an incentive to demonstrate how you value their time.

PATTI: It is also important to not be the 'only one' in such a group. I think one of the biggest potential pitfalls in this is tokenism – the idea of involving particular people so that you can say 'we have one of those.' It's also extremely important for me to know that other survivors will be advisory members. For example, when we go around at the beginning of the OBCCRI advisory committee meetings and people talk about what they're doing and there's an opportunity to say, 'things aren't going so well for me' or 'I'm going through the treatment with a friend of mine,' then I know that as a cancer survivor, that experience resonates. I appreciate the opportunity to have that included in the discussion at the beginning of the advisory meeting, but also, the pressure of being the only person in the room who might have that type of experience is dissipated. Having another cancer survivor there is helpful for checking things out to say 'well this isn't really true for me, is it true for you?' So I would just say that a question for an emerging research committee is: How do you support survivors either through resources or by eliminating the opportunity for tokenism?

COMMON VOICE: SUMMING UP

Being part of an advisory group and taking part in new research directions can feel a bit like being thrown back into the trenches – another version of the war against cancer and the struggle for life. However, it is not trenches, but boardrooms, focus groups, service delivery systems, art-based therapies, new research modalities, better knowledge translation, more targeted funding, better training through university and other curricula, and, of course, more advisory groups that are some of the current points of focus for change efforts in cancer care.

Importantly, the advisory process must be able to support and champion diversity and difference from within the advisory committee, just as researchers hope to do in their research choices, methods, and knowledge exchange strategies. It is crucial that tokenism according to particular facets of identity – for instance, race or sexual orientation – be circumvented by recognizing that each woman has multiple identities (Bradshaw & Inglis, 2004). We would also caution that survivorship itself is not a static category, and may not be a central realm of identity for everyone. As we move nearer to or further from our experiences with cancer, our perspectives shift, just as the landscape of cancer care changes and social attitudes are transformed over time. We need to be aware of the time and place in which we are working, and of diverse individual and community locations in cancer research, care, and experiential trajectories.

For the three of us, the experience of working with an innovative, evolving, visionary group of researchers has been timely and positive. We do very much want to caution, however, that this type of work is effortful and challenging. It is essential that supports for survivors are in place and that survivors assess their ability and energy regarding participation. When people come to a research advisory process from various perspectives and experiences, it is important to acknowledge this diversity. For instance, we all have personal and professional lives outside the research, which are often intertwined with our research interests and our reasons for being at the advisory table. Those reasons are often much more than academic, for survivors and researchers alike. We are all striving to keep the research grounded and relevant to lived experiences, healthcare practices, and social realities.

Acknowledgments

LESBIANS AND BREAST CANCER: A PARTICIPATORY RESEARCH PROJECT
The Project Team: Maureen Aslin, Jennifer Alexander, Lisa Barnoff, Pauline Bradbrook, Michèle Clarke, Teri Henderson, Pam Grassau, Patti McGillicuddy, Fran Odette, Samantha Sarra, Chris Sinding, Anna Travers, Danielle Vandezande
Women who participated in the study: Lillian, Mary Lou, Marcia, Kate, Sarah, Rosalie, Maureen, Paula, Paddy, Pauline, Jessica, Paula K., Glenda, Constance, Sherry, Liz, Teagan, Gerrie, Marie, Jacquie, Jann, Lou, Bonnie, Theresa, Laura, Anette
Partner Agencies: The 519 Church Street Community Centre, DAWN Ontario: DisAbled Women's Network Ontario, The Coalition for Lesbian & Gay Rights in Ontario, Gilda's Club, The Metropolitan Community Church of Toronto, The Ontario Breast Cancer Community Research Initiative, The Rainbow Health Network, Sherbourne Health Centre, Sunnybrook & Women's College Health Sciences Centre – Social Work & Professional Advisory Committee, Willow Breast Cancer Support & Resource Services
   This project was funded by the Canadian Breast Cancer Foundation, Ontario Chapter.

OLDER WOMEN WITH BREAST OR GYNECOLOGICAL CANCER STUDY
Principal Investigator: Chris Sinding
The Project Team: Jane Aronson, McMaster University, Pam Board and Barb Daize, Breast Cancer Support Services, Ann Wray Hampson and Wanda Risso, Thelma McGillivray, Older Women's Network, Jennifer Wiernikowski, Hamilton Regional Cancer Centre
   The Older Women's Project is one of three projects in the Intersecting Vulnerabilities research program, which was funded by the Canadian Institutes of Health Research. The Canadian Breast Cancer Foundation, Ontario Chapter funds the Ontario Breast Cancer Community Research Initiative, home of the Intersecting Vulnerabilities research program. The Older Women study was also supported by a grant from McMaster University.

LADIES IN WAITING? LIFE AFTER BREAST CANCER STUDY
Principal Investigator: Ross Gray
The Project Team, Advisors: Chris Sinding, Vrenia Ivonoffski, Ann Wray Hampson, Pamela Grassau, Falia Damianakis, Patti McGil-

licuddy, Wendy Arnold, Juliana Soares, Deborah Cauz, Margaret De-Gregorio, Dvora Levinson, Patricia Bower, Carole Keys, Sharyn Little

Ladies in Waiting? was developed by the Ontario Breast Cancer Community Research Initiative and Act II Studio at Ryerson University. Funding for *Ladies in Waiting?* was generously provided by the Canadian Breast Cancer Foundation, Ontario Chapter.

NOTES

1 The OBCCRI was formed out of a partnership between the Centre for Research in Women's Health, the Psychosocial and Behavioural Research Unit in the Toronto Sunnybrook Regional Cancer Centre at Sunnybrook Health Sciences Centre in Toronto, Ontario, and was funded by the Canadian Breast Cancer Foundation, Ontario Chapter. It was mandated to study the psychosocial needs of marginalized or underrepresented communities of women with breast cancer using participatory action research as one of its methodologies.
2 *Ladies in Waiting? Life after Breast Cancer* was a theatre production created from research transcripts by the researchers at the Ontario Breast Cancer Community Research Initiative and was toured.

REFERENCES

Bradshaw, P., & Inglis, S. (July, 2004). Diversity on nonprofit boards: Rethinking traditional frameworks through examining the emerging fringe. Paper presented at the Community of Inquiry Symposium, *Facing current realities: New knowledge in the Canadian voluntary sector*, Toronto, Ryerson University.

Brown, P., & Zavestoski, S. (2004). Social movements in health: An introduction. *Sociology of Health & Illness, 26*, 679–94.

Canadian Advisory Council on the Status of Women. (1995). What women prescribe: Report and recommendations. From the National Symposium *Women in partnership: Working towards inclusive, gender-sensitive health policies*.

Fine, M. (1994). Working the hyphens: Reinventing self and other in qualitative research. In N.K. Denzin & Y.S. Lincoln (Eds.), *Handbook of qualitative research* (pp. 70–82). Thousand Oaks, CA: Sage.

Gunaratnam, Y. (2003). *Researching 'race' and ethnicity: Methods, knowledge, and power*. London: Sage.

Hagen, N., & Whylie, B. (1998). Putting clinical practice guidelines into the hands of cancer patients. Editorial. *Canadian Medical Association Journal, 158*, 347–8.

Hagey, R.S. (1997). Guest editorial: The use and abuse of participatory action research. *Chronic Diseases in Canada, 18*(1). Retrieved August 21, 2007, from http://www.phac-aspc.gc.ca/publicat/cdic-mcc/18-1/a_e.html

Jones, S. (2002). (Re)writing the word: Methodological strategies and issues in qualitative research. *Journal of College Student Development, 43*, 461–73.

Klawiter, M. (2004). Breast cancer in two regimes: The impact of social movements on illness experience. *Sociology of Health and Illness, 26*, 845–74.

Minkler, M. (2004). Ethical challenges for the 'outside' researcher in community-based participatory research. *Health Education & Behavior, 31*, 684–97.

Porter, J., Parsons, S., & Robertson, C. (2006). Time for review: Supporting the work of an advisory group. *Journal of Research in Special Educational Needs, 6*(1), 11–16.

Sinding, C., & Cohen, M. (March 1996). *Changing concepts in women's health.* Canada-USA women's health forum commissioned paper, Ottawa. Retrieved August 17, 2007, from http://www.hc-sc.gc.ca/hl-vs/pubs/women-femmes/can-usa/back-promo_a_e.html

Yoshihama, M., & Carr, E.S. (2002). Community participation reconsidered: Feminist participatory action research with Hmong women. *Journal of Community Practice, 10*(4), 85–103.

PART FIVE

Implications and Impacts of Knowledge

11 Making a Difference with Research

CHRIS SINDING, JUDY GOULD, AND ROSS GRAY

The Ontario Breast Cancer Community Research Initiative (OBCCRI) was established to explore the psychosocial needs of marginalized women with breast cancer. Unlike most research units, however, our mandate extends beyond study: we have a stated commitment to increasing the responsiveness of health professionals and communities to the needs of the women with whom we work.

According to the usual ways of assessing researchers and research initiatives (publications generated, research dollars secured, research capacity built) OBCCRI is doing just fine. But over five years of developing, implementing, and sharing knowledge from research projects, have we really made a difference?

Certainly we have strategies and mechanisms in place for facilitating change:

- *Research is done in collaboration with people with cancer and cancer care professionals.* Like other researchers working towards social justice, we often adopt participatory approaches involving people most implicated in the research in project design and implementation. In addition to making the research questions more relevant and the research process smarter, involving survivors and professionals means that the findings we generate have champions in the real world, people involved who can make the findings directly relevant to a particular clinical or community context and encourage their uptake.
- *Research findings are presented directly to cancer survivors*, at community gatherings and cancer survivor-directed workshops and conferences.

- *Research findings are presented directly to health professionals* at cancer centre seminars and professional conferences.
- *Research findings are presented directly to health system administrators,* who have a role in changing policies that affect people with cancer.
- *Research findings are presented via user-friendly communication tools.* Our results are included in community organizations' newsletters and websites, on-line bulletins and institutionally-based newsletters and websites. We also produce and distribute booklets and reports summarizing our research.
- *Research findings are communicated creatively.* We have been among the pioneers of arts-based research dissemination (particularly research-based drama (Gray & Sinding, 2002)), joining the small but growing ranks of researchers who believe that qualitative studies are often best represented and received in narrative or imaginative forms.

We have attended, then, to the key factors that support change-making with research: the research itself, user engagement in the research, and strategies to increase impact (Nutley, Davies, Walter, & Wilkinson, 2004). We've tailored our findings to audiences and made them accessible – strategies known to increase the potential for change in practice and policy (Davies, Nutley, & Walter, 2005).

Yet from the first days of our research unit we talked about our accountability to the people who 'Run for the Cure' – the breast cancer survivors, family members, friends, and allies who raise the money that funds our research unit. Have we made a difference to them? And if we have, what kind of a difference is it?

Below we offer two vignettes – stories of two research projects, the knowledge-sharing strategies they employed, and the difference-making we perceive and claim for them. We then turn our attention to the phenomenon of 'knowledge translation' (KT), drawing forward cautions and opportunities for KT suggested by our work.

Nothing Fit Me: A Report about the Needs of Young Women with Breast Cancer

In the fall of 2001 the staff from the Canadian Breast Cancer Network (CBCN) and researchers from the Ontario Breast Cancer Community Research Initiative (OBCCRI) met to formulate a research plan to investigate the information and support experiences of young women who live with breast cancer. The CBCN describes itself as 'the network and voice of breast cancer survivors.' Its goals include supporting and informing Canadians concerned about breast cancer, promoting education and awareness about breast cancer, and ensuring that Canadians who have had a breast cancer diagnosis can attempt to influence research and healthcare policy (Canadian Breast Cancer Network, 2005).

Until this research project, little was known about the experiences of young Canadian women with breast cancer. Young women make up 22 per cent of all breast cancer survivors (Canadian Cancer Society / National Cancer Institute of Canada, 2005), and advocates and researchers were worried that their experiences had not been suitably documented or their needs appropriately addressed.

To begin this investigation, sixty-five young women were recruited to participate in ten focus groups, co-lead by CRI researchers. All women had been diagnosed with breast cancer at or before forty-five years of age. During the consultations the women were asked to discuss their information and support needs, current resources, and resource recommendations related to their diagnosis, treatment, and survivorship.

The focus group data was analysed and findings written up by CRI researchers. While a paper was written for an academic audience (Gould, Grassau, Gray, & Fitch, 2006) the more important version was collected in a report CRI researchers wrote for wide public distribution entitled *'Nothing Fit Me': The Information and Support Needs of Canadian Young Women with Breast Cancer* (Gould, James, Manthorne, Gray, & Fitch, 2002). This report revealed young women's perceptions that information, support, and programs / services did not 'fit' or match their age or life-stage. Missing information concerned, for example, the effects of adjuvant therapies on fertility, the signs and side effects of early menopause, how to relate to themselves and others sexually and intimately following treatment, and how to talk to their children about their cancer. The participants discussed the difficulty of affording unanticipated treatment-related expenses and of having the financial latitude to stay home from work immediately following treatment in order to facilitate recovery. Even within the cancer care system the women spoke about 'not fitting' into the profile of a typical breast cancer patient.

The young women recommended that breast cancer information match their age and life-stage and that healthcare providers create and implement workshops concerning, for example, sexuality, dating, and financial assistance. Regarding support, the women were adamant that efforts continue to be made to connect young women with breast can-

Table 10

> **YOUNG WOMEN WITH BREAST CANCER**
>
> ### Why was the research completed?
> The few studies exploring the experience of breast cancer for young women have illuminated issues, such as how women cope with the 'untimeliness' of the diagnosis; early menopause; impaired sexuality; and the effect of the diagnosis on their loved ones. In 2001, there was a paucity of Canadian research about the experience of breast cancer for young women.
>
> ### What methods were used?
> In partnership with the Canadian Breast Cancer Network (CBCN), the OBCCRI facilitated ten day-long consultations with sixty-five young women in five cities across Canada. All women had been diagnosed with breast cancer at or before forty-five years of age. During the consultations the women were asked to discuss their information and support experiences and needs, as well as resource recommendations related to their diagnosis, treatment, and survivorship.
>
> ### What were the key findings?
> - The overarching theme, 'Nothing Fit Me,' revealed that accessed information, support, and programs/services did not 'fit' or match the women's age or life-stage.
> - The first supporting theme illuminated that concerns about, for example, fertility, early menopause, breast reconstruction, sexuality, and mental health were not well addressed in the cancer literature or by health professionals.
> - The second supporting theme alluded to difficulties associated with communicating about cancer to children and in intimate relationships.
> - The final supporting theme focused on the difficulty of affording unanticipated treatment-related expenses.
> - Participants recommended that information and support match their age and life-stage and that health professionals create and implement several topical workshops concerning, for example, sexuality, lymphedema, and breast reconstruction.
>
> ### What are some implications or results of the research?
> The report 'Nothing Fit Me' written about these findings and made available on the CBCN website changed practice in the following ways:

- a menopause clinic for women catapulted into premature menopause was created at the Hamilton Regional Cancer Centre
- in the Locally Advanced Breast Cancer Clinic at Toronto-Sunnybrook Regional Cancer Centre (TSRCC), pre-menopausal women now have the option at intake of referral to the fertility clinic
- a group therapy program was developed at TSRCC's Locally Advanced Breast Clinic (LABC) where young women with breast cancer make up a large proportion of that clinic's population
- OBCCRI is working in partnership with the LABC clinic at TSRCC, Wellspring, and Willow Breast Cancer Support and Resource Services to implement a one on one peer support service for young women.

cer through either community- or hospital-based support groups, or one-to-one peer counselling either face to face or by a telephone hotline. The following has occurred since the report was made public.

STAKEHOLDERS CAME TOGETHER FOR ACTION PLANNING:

- CBCN used the report to guide the National Strategy and Action Plan for Young Women with Breast Cancer and the first advocacy workshop with and for young women with breast cancer (in partnership with Willow, a national breast cancer information and support organization).
- The report was used to justify the first national conference on young women with breast cancer.

CLINICAL AND POLICY CHANGES WERE MADE:

- At Toronto-Sunnybrook Regional Cancer Centre:
  - Intake procedures have changed: pre-menopausal women now have the option of referral to a fertility clinic
  - A group therapy program was developed that predominantly serves young women with breast cancer
  - A Young Women's Clinic has been proposed
- At another regional cancer centre in southern Ontario, a menopause clinic was created for women catapulted into premature menopause as a result of breast cancer treatment.
- Efforts have been undertaken between OBCCRI and three partner

organizations to implement a one on one peer support service for younger women with breast cancer.
• The CBCN is planning workshops, a hotline, and the development of clinical practice guidelines.

The sentence that precedes the bullet points above, 'the following has occurred since the report was made public,' masks two realities. First, it hides the reality that some of these events and changes in policy and practice are direct outcomes of the research and the *Nothing Fit Me* report, while others are less clearly linked. Second, it hides the agency and effort of individuals – and perhaps more importantly the *relationships* – that made it all happen.

Establishing cause-and-effect relationships between any particular study and policy or practice change is notoriously difficult (Davies et al., 2005). We know for certain that the creation of a National Strategy for Young Women in Canada launched by the CBCN and the CBCN/Willow advocacy workshop emerged directly from the report. In fact, the research and development of the report were required as justification and direction for these two initiatives. Our research team knew about these initiatives mainly because we were invited to present the data at the National Strategy and Action Plan for Young Women stakeholder meeting and because our partners at CBCN informed us about the advocacy workshop. This certainly aids the ability to track the impact of the knowledge we have generated!

Yet even when research has a direct impact, researchers may not know about it. Over two years after the *Nothing Fit Me* report was made available, two advanced practice nurses informally told the principal investigator how they had come upon the report and immediately instituted change in their cancer centres. One nurse recalled that a breast cancer patient told her about the report. She called CBCN for a copy, read it, and implemented the routine offer of referral to fertility counselling for women in her clinic. The other nurse recollected reading a community-based newsletter in which we had communicated the project findings. She emailed CBCN for a copy and, after reading the report, created the menopause clinic mentioned above. Both of these nurses later participated as advisory members on other OBCCRI projects.

We learned of other outcomes even less directly. For example, a colleague passed along the *Young and the Breastless* conference advertisement and on the cover of that abstract were paraphrased quotes from the report justifying the need for the conference. Another colleague picked up a national magazine and found an article about young women and breast cancer that made reference to the *Nothing Fit Me* report.

Among the many things that have become clear to us over the past five years is the centrality of relationships to ensuring research makes a difference. Influencing policies and practices depends on sustained relationships with decision-makers (Lomas, 2000). It has been critical for OBCCRI to establish an organizational presence in the breast cancer and health research communities, and to develop linkages to a wide variety of community and professional organizations and individuals. Relationship-building and the work required to solidify these relationships (such as presenting research at stakeholder meetings, participating as members of advisory committees poised to implement research) have been cornerstones of our work. Relationships – both intentionally created, and emerging from our 'hanging around' in the breast cancer community – have facilitated the uptake of our research; it is also through our relationships that we know what we know about the difference we have made.

Ladies in Waiting? A Drama about Life after Breast Cancer

Aware that the experiences and needs of longer-term cancer survivors are not much explored, members of our research team interviewed women who were four years or more beyond a breast cancer diagnosis about their information needs. In the article published from the research (Gray et al., 1998) we offered recommendations for policy and practice. We also created a booklet for survivors, highlighting key study findings and describing resources (cancer agencies, books, websites, and so on) that spoke to the gaps in information research participants had identified.

Yet while both efforts to 'make a difference' with this study made good sense, neither felt sufficient. So much of what survivors had said in interviews went missing in the 'translation' of their narratives into recommendations. While we had carefully selected resources for the booklet to reflect the information needs survivors had identified, the booklet failed to speak to the sources, meaning, and life consequences of those needs.

So we undertook a collaboration with Act II Studio, a theatre school for adults over age fifty at Ryerson University in Toronto, Ontario. Under the leadership of Act II's artistic director, Vrenia Ivonoffski, a

Table 11

LADIES IN WAITING? LIFE AFTER BREAST CANCER

Why was the research completed?
The issues facing long-term survivors of breast cancer have been
relatively neglected, with most health system attention being focused on
women who require active treatment for disease. Various cancer support
and advocacy organizations have called for improved understanding of
survivors' needs. This study was requested by members of the Ontario
Breast Cancer Information Exchange Partnership, a coalition of organizations working together to improve access to information and support
for women affected by breast cancer.

What methods were used?
We conducted nine focus groups around Ontario with women at least
four years beyond a breast cancer diagnosis.

What were the key findings?
Women discussed the ongoing impact of their initial disease experience
and described continued uncertainty about possible recurrence, a lack
of information, and concerns about communication with professionals.
(For details, see Gray et al., 1998.)

What are some implications or results of the research?
Buoyed by the success of two previous research-based dramas,
OBCCRI researchers undertook a third collaboration with Act II Studio,
a theatre school for adults over age fifty at Ryerson University. Artistic
director Vrenia Ivonoffski provided leadership to the script development team (SDT), which included members of the research team along
with ten cancer survivors. Members of the SDT read the focus group
transcripts and participated in a series of meetings to explore themes
in the transcripts. Drawing on the work generated by the script development team, Ivonoffski wrote *Ladies in Waiting?* (Ivonoffski, 2002). The
script was reviewed by members of the team, performed before a test
audience of researchers, health professionals, and cancer survivors,
and then revised. It was performed live for four audiences composed
mainly of survivors and their family members and friends in urban and
suburban settings. A video was then created from the drama, screened
in four communities in suburban Ontario and at the World Breast Cancer

Conference in British Columbia, Canada, and mailed to cancer support organizations across the country.

See references at end of chapter for sources.

script development team (ten cancer survivors along with members of the original research team) read study transcripts and participated in a series of half-day meetings to explore themes in the transcripts, drawing on their own personal experiences and engaging in a series of improvisation exercises. Working from the research transcripts and the images and dialogue generated by the team, Ivonoffski wrote *Ladies in Waiting? Life After Breast Cancer* (Ivonoffski, 2002) as a drama that reveals breast cancer's physically and emotionally chronic nature. The drama directly challenges dominant social messages that cancer is or should be 'over' soon after treatment has ended. It conveys women's persistent awareness of profoundly changed bodies, the ongoing consequences of treatment, and, critically, women's knowledge that cancer might recur. The knowledge that cancer might recur underpins several dramatic scenes – scenes where women work to interpret bodily signs and try to plan for the future, struggling with low-level anxiety and intermittent acute fear. In *Ladies in Waiting?* the experience of life after a breast cancer diagnosis is juxtaposed, often with humour, against a public discourse that sets up cancer survivorship as a kind of achievement. The drama was performed in Toronto and captured on video; the video was screened in several Ontario communities, and then mailed to over five-hundred groups and agencies that serve women with breast cancer.

Ladies in Waiting? is 'out there.' Yet the fact of its wide dissemination tells us very little about the effects it has had on people's lives. So we distributed questionnaires to audience members (drawing both quantitative and qualitative data) and recorded discussions between the people who hosted the drama, audience members, and researchers.

Almost four hundred audience members returned questionnaires about *Ladies in Waiting?* The vast majority – over 90 per cent – agreed or strongly agreed that they benefited from seeing the production, and a similar percentage said they would recommend it for others. Written comments suggested that the drama offered a mirror of experience, reducing isolation and normalizing the struggles of survivorship. Other comments suggested that the drama offered insights about survivorship for family and friends, increasing understanding and empathy.

These are all important outcomes. If the research team had defined desired outcomes for *Ladies in Waiting?* these would have been high on our list. Yet as we continued to review feedback forms from audience members, something more emerged. We were struck by how frequently survivors and those around them suggested that the knowledge about survivorship contained in *Ladies in Waiting?* is not readily available in the cancer community – or, even further, that this knowledge is 'covered up.' It became clear that the effects of *Ladies in Waiting?* must be understood is this context – and, it became clear that in this context, the drama had more and different benefits than we had initially recognized.

For instance, many audience members suggested that *Ladies in Waiting?* offered rare access to the social and emotional worlds of survivors. Relatives and friends described the drama as 'a wide awakening and learning process of what is experienced,' and 'an eye-opener.' An audience member wrote, 'My dearest friend is a breast cancer survivor. I have tried to be a support and encouragement. I realize now what she has been facing, but could not express. Thank you for opening this door.' A survivor and activist praised *Ladies in Waiting?* saying 'it's the way we would like to be able to tell it.'

The idea that survivors have not been able to tell their stories in the ways they would wish can imply that images and language for describing life in the years after a cancer diagnosis are not readily available. This analysis is supported by Little, Paul, Jordens, and Sayers (2002, p. 176) who contend that society has yet to create an adequate discourse of cancer survivorship:

> The survivor has as yet no specially defined status, no modes of performance that are socially validated. The survivor can therefore fit only into pre-existent and inadequate paradigms of the normal or the chronically ill, into metaphors of the victim or the hero ... the experience of the survivor awaits articulation and affirmation, in a discourse that recognizes the adhesiveness of the extreme experience, and the cognitive, emotional, physical and moral tensions that are part of survivorship.

In some way, then, we can understand *Ladies in Waiting?* as responding to Little and colleagues' call for the 'articulation and affirmation' of the experience of the survivor, as providing – in an accessible way

– accurate and sympathetic language and images where few have been available.

Yet the absence of a discourse of cancer survivorship is only one way to account for the lack of understanding in the cancer community and beyond about cancer's chronicity. Audience members suggest, in fact, that the truths of survivorship contained in *Ladies in Waiting?* are often 'covered up,' both by survivors and those around them. In these narratives, it is not that images and language are unavailable; it is that survivors cannot or do not reveal their experiences. One survivor who saw the production said, for instance, that the most helpful aspect of it was 'women talking about what we think of, only don't speak of.' An exchange after a screening unfolded as follows:

AUDIENCE MEMBER: [The video] is something our family and friends should see. It sums up perfectly those thoughts and feelings.
FACILITATOR: What is it about this that you want family and friends to see?
AUDIENCE MEMBER: The things you don't tell them.

While survivors sometimes perceived benefits to themselves from muting or containing the struggles of survivorship, they more commonly referred to various kinds of social pressure to be 'over' cancer. '[Survivors] are very encouraged to put this behind them,' noted one woman. 'It's poignant, once surgery/ treatment are done, people around you feel, "fine, now you are done with it, and you can move on," but it doesn't go away,' said another. Cancer funding agencies were implicated by one viewer: 'I hate the "cancer can be beaten" message. It's still a horrible disease. Yet there is this message that everything will be fine.' 'People ask you how you are feeling, and you are supposed to say "I'm fine" – and you're not,' one woman said from the audience. 'I keep telling myself I belong to the liar's club,' she continued, to laughter.

The context of the 'cover up' of survivors' experiences allow us to understand some of the more complex and subtle outcomes of *Ladies in Waiting?* In the course of responding to the production, survivors articulated a set of entitlements – entitlements to their own experiences, to confirmation of survivorship's ongoing-ness by people around them, and to freedom from the pressure to hide their experience. The production spoke to one survivor, for instance, of 'the importance of not minimizing the diagnosis to myself and others.' Another woman responded to a question about the most helpful parts of the production with the following: 'I will never be "over" this disease and others need to recognize I can't totally forget it.' In this statement, a survivor calls for – demands, even – recognition for the enormity of breast cancer's impact on her life, from the people around her.

Not everyone watching *Ladies in Waiting?* spoke about it in glowing terms. Some women, for instance, said they found it 'depressing.' Yet accompanying such assessments were comments such as 'it hit home.' The drama's sometimes difficult impact was, it seems, part and parcel of its resonance with audience members' experiences. The association of distress with negative evaluations of the production, or a desire not to have seen it, was extremely rare. Some audience members spoke, in fact, of the merits of being upset. More commonly, viewers who acknowledged they had been upset by the production affirmed, unprompted, the production's realistic portrayal of survivorship (Sinding, Gray, Grassau, Damianakis, & Hampson, 2006).

The kind of analysis presented here, of the complex and layered effects of *Ladies in Waiting?* is not quickly or easily generated. That the production offered benefits was evident from responses to standardized questions. Yet the nature of the benefits, the subtler benefits, and the ways benefit can occur even when (in this case some might say, because) the research-sharing vehicle is 'depressing' – these can only be understood from survivors' narratives, and through sustained conversation between survivors and researchers. Here again the crucial role of relationships – of knowledge *exchange* (Lomas, 2000) between researchers and their audiences – is apparent.

The KT (Knowledge Translation) Bandwagon, and Our Place on It

When OBCCRI researchers first crafted our mission and goals we affirmed a commitment to sharing research knowledge with a range of audiences, using a broad spectrum of strategies. At the time we were only dimly aware of the phenomenon called 'knowledge translation' (KT). The Canadian Institutes of Health Research (2005) has recently defined knowledge translation as:

> the exchange, synthesis and ethically-sound application of knowledge – within a complex system of interactions among researchers and users – to accelerate the capture of the benefits of research for Canadians through improved health, more effective services and products, and a strengthened health care system.

As KT continues to gain momentum, we are called upon to assess its congruence and points of discord with our own beliefs and approaches.

Current enthusiasm for knowledge translation links with broad trends to rationalize research and health service provision. Research advocates and funding bodies are increasingly pressed to justify the resources directed to research (Nutley et al., 2004). At the other end of the spectrum, health professionals and decision-makers are increasingly called to justify, with research, their interventions (Rycroft-Malone et al., 2004). (For a critique of the movement towards evidence-based practice, see Davies, 2003; Holloway, 2001; Larner, 2004.)

Efforts to render research and its uptake more accountable and efficient are usually seen as entirely laudable. Yet as Baines (2007) points out, in the current political context 'accountability' often means a return on investment for taxpayers, rather than accountability to research participants, marginalized groups, or the collective of citizens.

Researchers have also raised concerns about how the current emphasis on knowledge translation may unfold in practice. Certain kinds of research – particularly basic research in the sciences and theoretical work in the social sciences – may go unsupported and unfunded because its effects on policy and practice are by nature unclear or haphazardly realized. As well, much social science research is about (contested) understandings of how the social world operates. The implications of such research are rarely distillable into clear policy and practice recommendations. Even when offered in creative and accessible forms, the effects of such research are not easily measured (Gray, Fitch, Labrecque, & Greenberg, 2003; Nutley et al., 2004). Some researchers worry that the 'problem of measurement' (including the lack of appropriate tools, and perhaps more importantly, the un-measurability of some change processes) will lead to an under-appreciation of much social science research, and many promising research sharing strategies.

To understand the potential and pitfalls of KT for our own work (and vice versa) we can draw from the vignettes above and spin out the metaphor of 'translation.'

The *Nothing Fit Me* report had a pre-established 'listener': an advocacy organization committed to taking up research findings and recommendations about young women and breast cancer in its own work. At the same time, our 'translation' was overheard: people we did not speak with but to whom we are proximate because of the networks we have developed had access to the report and were able to act on it. In assessing research impact, then, we must remain aware that our research may have positive outcomes that we simply do not know about.

Proponents of KT encourage researchers to spell out the policy implications of their work and to evaluate their efforts at knowledge translation. We are not averse to such efforts – far from it. But as the *Ladies in Waiting?* project makes clear, certain kinds of knowledge defy 'recommendation,' and certain benefits of knowledge translation defy any standardized evaluation. While *Ladies in Waiting?* was taken up by cancer survivors mostly as we had hoped, it also translated in ways we never could have anticipated: 'fostering survivor entitlement' was not among the outcomes we defined or imagined. As Davies and colleagues (2005, p. 13) put it, 'research can contribute not only to decisional *choices,* but also to the formation of *values,* the creation of new *understandings and possibilities,* and to the quality of public and professional *discourse and debate*' (emphasis in original). Knowing this, we must take care to avoid privileging the most instrumental and readily identifiable research impacts, or the most (apparently) cost-effective and validated knowledge translation strategies.

OBCCRI researchers claim our seats on the KT bandwagon with care. Our interests lie in more abundant (rather than leaner) definitions of what counts as research and as knowledge translation, and in more flexible and creative (rather than more standardized) ways of understanding and assessing research impact. We concur with Baines's (2007) assessment that social justice agendas are best served when 'making a difference' is integral to the research enterprise. In this regard Baines encourages attention to Lather's (1986, p. 67) 'catalytic validity,' a revaluation of research projects based on the 'degree to which the research process re-orients, focuses, and energizes participants in what Freire (1973) terms "conscientization," knowing reality in order to better transform it.'

And, as always, we circle back to relationships. Relationships with research participants, community members, and decision-makers enable the uptake of research findings; they also maximize the number and kinds of people who will 'overhear' and make use of our research. Knowledge about relationships, as an outcome of much social science research, may require 'translating' in ways and settings quite outside those commonly recommended in the KT literature. Finally, relationships allow us to know much more fully than we might otherwise the nature and quality of the ripples our research makes in the world.

Acknowledgments

LADIES IN WAITING? LIFE AFTER BREAST CANCER STUDY
Principal Investigator: Ross Gray
The Project Team, Advisors: Chris Sinding, Vrenia Ivonoffski, Ann Wray Hampson, Pamela Grassau, Falia Damianakis, Patti McGillicuddy, Wendy Arnold, Juliana Soares, Deborah Cauz, Margaret DeGregorio, Dvora Levinson, Patricia Bower, Carole Keys, Sharyn Little
Ladies in Waiting? was developed by the Ontario Breast Cancer Community Research Initiative and Act II Studio at Ryerson University. Funding for Ladies in Waiting? was generously provided by the Canadian Breast Cancer Foundation, Ontario Chapter.

YOUNG WOMEN WITH BREAST CANCER PROJECT
Principal Investigator: Judy Gould
The Project Team: Pamela Grassau, Jackie Manthorne, Ross Gray, Marg Fitch
This project was funded by the Community Capacity Building arm of the Canadian Breast Cancer Initiative of Health Canada. In-kind resources were provided by the Ontario Breast Cancer Community Research Initiative, which is funded by the Canadian Breast Cancer Foundation, Ontario Chapter.

REFERENCES

Baines, D. (2007). The case for catalytic validity: Building health and safety through knowledge transfer. *Policy and Practice in Health and Safety, 5*(1), 75–89.
Canadian Breast Cancer Network. (2005). *About CBCN*. Retrieved December 2005, from http://www.cbcn.ca/
Canadian Cancer Society/ National Cancer Institute of Canada. (2005). *Canadian cancer statistics 2005*. Toronto, Canada.
Canadian Institutes of Health Research. (2005). *About knowledge translation*. Retrieved December, 2005, from http://www.cihr-irsc.gc.ca/e/29418.html
Davies, B. (2003). Death to critique and dissent? The policies and practices of

new managerialism and of 'evidence-based practice.' *Gender and Education,* *15*(1), 91–103.

Davies, H., Nutley, S., & Walter, I. (2005). *Approaches to assessing the non-aca-* *demic impact of social science research: Report of the Economic and Social Research* *Council symposium 12–13 May 2005.* University of St Andrews, Scotland: Research Unit for Research Utilisation.

Freire, P. (1973). *Pedagogy of the oppressed.* New York: Seabury Press.

Gould, J., Grassau, P., Gray, R., & Fitch, M. (2006). 'Nothing fit me': Nation- wide consultations with young women with breast cancer. *Health Expecta-* *tions, 9*(2), 158–73.

Gould, J., James, P., Manthorne, J., Gray, R., & Fitch, M. (2002). *'Nothing fit me':* *The information and support needs of Canadian young women with breast cancer.* Retrieved December 2005, from http://www.cbcn.ca/english/publications. php?display&en&22

Gray, R., Fitch, M., Greenberg, M., Hampson, A., Doherty, M., & Labrecque, M. (1998). The information needs of well, longer-term survivors of breast cancer. *Patient Education and Counseling, 44,* 245–55.

Gray, R., Fitch, M., Labrecque, M., & Greenberg, M. (2003). Reactions of health professionals to a research-based theatre production. *Journal of Cancer Educa-* *tion, 18*(4), 223–9.

Gray, R.E., Greenberg, M., Fitch, M., Sawka, C., Hampson, A., Labrecque, M., et al. (1998). Information needs of women with metastatic breast cancer. *Cancer Prevention and Control, 2*(2), 57–62.

Gray, R., & Sinding, C. (2002). *Standing ovation: Performing social science research* *about cancer.* Walnut Creek, CA: AltaMira Press.

Holloway, W. (2001). The psycho-social subject in EBP. *Journal of Social Work* *Practice, 15*(1), 9–22.

Ivonoffski, V. (2002). *Ladies in waiting? A play about life after breast cancer.* To- ronto Sunnybrook Regional Cancer Centre.

Larner, G. (2004). Family therapy and the politics of evidence. *Journal of Family* *Therapy, 26*(1), 17–39.

Lather, P. (1986). Issues of validity in openly ideological research: Between a rock and a soft place. *Interchange, 17*(4), 63–84.

Little, M., Paul, K., Jordens, C., & Sayers, E.J. (2002). Survivorship and dis- courses of identity. *Psycho-Oncology, 11,* 170–8.

Lomas, J. (2000). Using 'linkage and exchange' to move research into policy at a Canadian foundation. *Health Affairs, 19*(3), 236–40.

Nutley, S., Davies, H., Walter, I., & Wilkinson, J. (2004). *Developing projects to* *assess research impact.* University of St Andrews: Research Unit for Research Utilisation.

Rycroft-Malone, J., Harvey, G., Seers, K., Kitson, A., McCormack, B., & Titchen, A. (2004). An exploration of the factors that influence the implementation of evidence into practice. *Journal of Clinical Nursing, 13,* 913–24.

Sinding, C., Gray, R., Grassau, P., Damianakis, F., & Hampson, A. (2006). Audience responses to a research-based drama about life after breast cancer. *Psycho-Oncology, 15,* 694–700.

12 Moving Knowledge: The Possibilities and Complexities of Qualitative and Participatory Research

MARGARET I. FITCH

The ultimate aim of research in health and illness is to uncover new knowledge that will aid in the improvement of patient care. To accomplish this, researchers must not only conduct the research and uncover the knowledge, but also share that knowledge so that healthcare providers and decision-makers have it available for use. For researchers who engage in qualitative and participatory approaches, a central challenge is finding the avenues for effective dissemination of their findings. This chapter will highlight some of the current thinking about knowledge dissemination and explore some of the learnings about it from work of the Ontario Breast Cancer Community Research Initiative (OBCCRI). It is my hope that other investigators engaged in this type of research will be able to build on the lessons in the work. Clearly, the knowledge uncovered through qualitative and participatory methods has the potential to improve patient care and needs to be incorporated in the processes of decision-making in healthcare.

One of the significant learnings emphasized throughout the work of the OBCCRI is that partnerships set the stage for sharing new knowledge. The involvement of patients and survivors created a wonderful initial step for disseminating the results of the research. Those who were involved in the planning and advisory groups of each research endeavour are a ready-made audience with whom to share findings. Many are members of community groups and are only too eager to have presentations given by the researchers at their meetings or gatherings. Some groups have newsletters or websites and see that the research results can also be shared through those avenues. Additionally, the members of OBCCRI have presented at professional and academic conferences regularly in the course of their work and written a variety of academic journal articles. These avenues are part of the traditional routes for sharing research findings. They reach a particular audience. However, these routes alone have little impact on the implementation based on the actual findings of the research of new approaches in policy or practice.

Hence, the larger question for me is one of how to move awareness of the results of qualitative and participatory research into the wider community and to have it actually impact the delivery of care and support for individuals living with cancer. Given the nature of the work, the type of data, and the messages that need to be communicated, how do the research results need to be shared to achieve effective uptake and utilization? If one embraces the idea that health-related research is done, at least in part, to influence decision-making, stimulate policy change, and improve approaches to patient care, this will not happen if the research results are not shared with the appropriate audiences in relevant and meaningful ways.

During our time together at OBCCRI we were exposed to just how complex this process of knowledge sharing really is – and how much research is needed on this topic itself. The process of sharing knowledge and having that knowledge picked up and used as the basis for decision-making is fraught with potential pitfalls. It is a process that requires concerted, focused effort if it is to be successful. Fortunately, interest in the topic is growing as recognition increases about the general uneven adoption of research findings into practice arenas. Particularly in cancer care, there is a wide gap between what is known and practised across the cancer care spectrum, which calls for enhanced knowledge dissemination and uptake (Grunfeld, Zitzelsberger, Hayter, Berman, Cameron, Evans, & Stern, 2004).

A Variety of Conceptualizations

In this section I will summarize some of the current thinking about the dissemination and uptake of research results. In later sections I will highlight some of the issues we learned about through our time with OBCCRI.

Currently there are a variety of conceptualizations about the process of sharing research information or knowledge and having it taken up and used by others. The Canadian Institutes of Health Research (CIHR) defines knowledge translation as 'the exchange, synthesis and ethically-sound application of research findings within a complex system of relationships among researchers and knowledge users' (CIHR, 2002). A more focused definition for knowledge translation is 'the effective and timely incorporation of evidence-based information into the practices of health professionals in such a way as to effect optimal health care outcomes and maximize the potential for the health system' (University of Toronto, as adapted from the CIHR definition, 2001).

Related terms include knowledge utilization (Landry, Amara, & Lamari, 2002), knowledge transfer (Eveland, 1986), knowledge mobilization (McCall, Rootman, & Bayley, 2005), knowledge exchange (Lomas, 1993), diffusion of innovations (Rogers, 2003), and knowledge use (Logan & Graham, 1998). Knowledge utilization refers to the use of research to guide practice. While it falls under the purview of 'evidence-based practice,' it is more specific to research evidence – the findings of scientific studies. Both knowledge utilization and evidence-based practice are broader than research utilization, encompassing the use of forms of evidence other than research evidence alone (Estabrooks, 1999).

Although all these terms are often used interchangeably (Grunfeld et al., 2004), each term has a slightly different emphasis on elements of the process that are considered to be of significance. For example, knowledge diffusion focuses on the rather passive process of simply getting the information out, while knowledge mobilization embraces the notion of motivating a target audience to action; knowledge exchange embraces the notion of a two-way exchange of information between knowledge generators and knowledge users, while knowledge utilization focuses on the actual uptake of knowledge and its use in practice.

Clearly, all conceptualizations embody the notion that there needs to be knowledge generation, knowledge sharing, and knowledge use (see fig. 12.1). Research has to be conducted and new knowledge produced. Once the knowledge has been uncovered, it needs to be shared with others who have the potential to make use of it. Once they are in possession of the 'new knowledge,' the users need to be able to actually utilize the knowledge or information. How each of these activities occurs has an influence on the eventual outcome of knowledge uptake and use.

There is a growing appreciation of the many factors that influence these processes, and several models that have been created to try to capture and illustrate the complexity (Lomas, 2000; Landry et al., 2002; Graham & Logan, 2004; Grol, 1997). Many of the models have similar aspects and no one model is considered superior to another at this point

Figure 12.1. Process of Knowledge Exchange or Transfer – Key Components

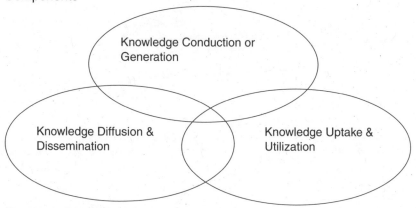

Knowledge Conduction or Generation

Knowledge Diffusion & Dissemination

Knowledge Uptake & Utilization

Fig. 12.1 by M.I. Fitch

in time. Originally, there was a sense that the process of knowledge translation was linear. The working assumption was that if the knowledge was made available, practitioners and policy makers would read it and use it. These models predominated in the 1960s to mid-1990s and made use of the language of dissemination, diffusion, transfer, and uptake. Knowledge was seen as a product that could be handed off to users and generalized for use across contexts (Best, 2006).

Relationship models emerged in the mid-1990s and focus on the notion of exchange. Here, knowledge is seen as coming from multiple sources, to be used within and through the context of social relationships and networks. It is also context-specific and needs to be adapted for use in local settings. That knowledge use is conceptualized as being embedded within social relationships is a major shift in thinking and has significant implications for sharing research knowledge and expecting it to be utilized.

Key influences in the knowledge exchange or translation process are depicted in a simple manner in figure 12.2. In the first place, an investigator needs to consider what the fundamental message is that needs to be communicated. Every message has levels of complexity inherent in the message as well as implications for the 'listener.' This message came home to me early in my nursing career when I worked in intensive care. A patient who was intubated and on a ventilator, unable to speak be-

Figure 12.2. Influences in Knowledge Exchange or Transfer Process

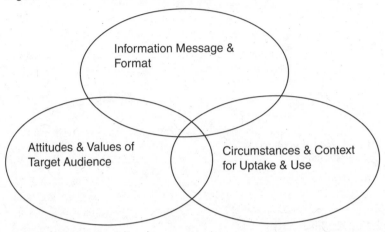

Fig. 12.2 by M.I. Fitch

cause of the endotracheal tube, could find a way to tell me he wanted to sit up, but telling me he wanted to see a certain person for a particular reason was more difficult or impossible given the limited channels of communication that were available at the time. A complex message, as well as the available venue and format for delivery, can hinder its successful sharing. Part of the challenge in communicating research results is to find the key message that needs to be communicated and make it as clear and easy to understand as possible.

The intended audience is another critical consideration, especially in terms of their attitudes and values. Attitudes and values will colour or influence the perception of any message. A particularly difficult message to deliver is one that states that patients would like something different than what they are currently receiving. Some healthcare professionals might react to this message as if it is a criticism of the care they are providing. Instead of being open to dialogue about change and improvement, they feel defensive and reluctant to change their practice approaches. This may be more likely if the healthcare professionals are feeling particularly overwhelmed with their patient caseloads or workloads. And, healthcare professionals' beliefs about how patients ought to behave may influence how open they will be to data that comes from patients – should patients be passive recipients of care or autonomous individuals with responsibility for decisions about the care of their own bodies? Recent work by Gabbey and le May (2004) emphasized the finding that 'clinicians rarely accessed, appraised, and used explicit evidence directly from research ... instead they relied on "mind-lines," collectively reinforced, internalized, tacit guidelines' (p. 1015). Breaking through those 'mind-lines' is a considerable challenge, especially in the cancer care environment of today, which can be described as one of escalating patient caseloads, increasing complexity of treatment protocols, and decreasing financial resources (Canadian Strategy in Cancer Control, 2004).

Finally, the context (environment, setting) in which one expects the new knowledge to be used, and how it is expected to be used, are of critical importance. For example, if using the knowledge means that extra time will be required for its application during a patient-provider interaction, and members of the healthcare team lose time in their day but do not see any gain for it, the use of knowledge will soon fall away (Grol & Grimshaw, 2003). If use of the knowledge means additional 'hassle' in the care delivery process, the knowledge could easily be set aside and not used, especially in an environment that is busy and chaotic (Blasi, Harkness, Ernst, Georgiou, & Kleijnen, 2001; Oxman, 1995). The intended users of the knowledge must have the capacity to make use of it in the way that was envisioned. Sometimes this will require education initiatives and changes in care delivery processes of the practice arena (Montague, 2006). Making use of new evidence may require the acquisition of new resources, facilities, and enhanced staff support.

Thinking about 'Use' of Evidence

What is actually meant by the term 'use'? When we say we expect that practitioners make use of research knowledge, what does that really mean? Being clear about the expected behaviour or practice change that would reflect use of a research result is an important consideration, especially in light of thinking about what constitutes 'success' of a knowledge exchange strategy or approach. We have been repeatedly challenged to think about this in our work within OBCCRI. When a new medication is developed and tested through clinical trial, use of that medication in practice with eligible patients is clear. However, the findings generated by the OBCCRI about the range of experiences breast cancer survivors had during their treatment could spark debate about how to make best use of that evidence.

An individual may read or hear new information and 'use' that information in a variety of ways. The information may help in providing new insight into a situation or a new way of conceptualizing an issue. It may provide validation that the approach they were already using in their practice was fine and they ought to continue. Or it may result in their incorporating new aspects to their assessment and intervention with patients. The actual use is, in some measure, also linked to the nature of the message. For example, practitioners might learn that young women with breast cancer often experience concerns about fertility, but unless there is an intervention available to offer, they may not investigate whether or not a particular patient is experiencing these concerns. In this instance, simply telling practitioners that there has been research revealing that young women experience distress about loss of fertility after breast cancer treatment might not result in a change in their practice. Revealing that there are interventions that could counteract that distress, if instituted before cancer treatments, is a different message and could have a different effect on changing practice.

On the other hand, practitioners who find out that fertility issues are common for young women living with breast cancer may use this information to support patients who are experiencing concerns by validating the patient's experience as normal and linking it to the experience of treatment. It could also be argued that different approaches in care will be utilized by different disciplines. What a physician does with the fertility information may be different from what a nurse or a social worker might do. Hence, the context, the message inherent in the research knowledge, and the actual players can have a significant impact on what is meant by 'use.'

Moving towards Knowledge Integration

As researchers have begun to pay more attention to how to move research results into practice and policy, and have observed the remaining gaps between knowledge and its use, they have begun to direct investigation towards understanding the various influences within the knowledge translation process. This has extended the perspective beyond the individual practitioner to a wider view of the system in which the practitioner works. Clearly, the process of knowledge exchange is complex (Larsen, 1980), interactive (Rogers, 2002), and reliant on the user's knowledge, beliefs, and experiences (NCDDR, 1996); multiple factors come into play in any one situation. But if we are to think about achieving successful utilization and sustainable change, attention needs to be given to a system level perspective.

Systems model thinking embraces the notion of knowledge integration (Best, 2006). The knowledge cycle is tightly woven within priorities, culture, and context; knowledge needs to be integrated to inform decision-making and policy; relationships within the organization mediate throughout the cycle, and the degree of use is a function of the integration of the organization and its system. The challenge is to think about knowledge synthesis in terms of a matrix with individual, team/organization, and system/policy on one axis, and basic, clinical, and population research knowledge on the other. What is needed to be successful with knowledge exchange for clinical knowledge at the individual level will be different from demands at the system level. Greenhalgh, Robert, MacFarlane, Bate, & Kyriakidou (2004) recently wrote a wonderful article describing what one needs to think about and focus on when trying to achieve effective knowledge exchange at these three levels.

For example, influencing practice change on the part of individuals has a great deal to do with individual personality traits, perception, and coping styles; influencing change at the team or organizational level is more about social networks and relationships, opinion leaders, incentives, and team skills; influencing systems or policy change is about champions, boundary spanners, formal programs, and an organization's capacity for innovation. However, at all levels, the evidence needs to be seen as credible, the message inherent in the evidence needs to be clear, and the topic needs to be of relevance to the target audience (i.e., help them solve a problem they are experiencing).

Researcher Role in Knowledge Translation or Exchange

As a researcher, one clearly needs to identify the message inherent in a new piece of research knowledge and understand who the audience is for that message. The delivery or communication of the message needs to be crafted for its intended audience and delivered in the appropriate format. The expectations for use of the information (i.e., how it will change practice or policy) need to be clearly articulated and attention paid to the potential barriers to practice change. Those barriers will need to be removed or altered if the expected outcome is to be achieved.

I question, however, whether a researcher can, or ought to be, involved in all of these steps or activities. It is a question that needs to be debated. And I would suggest that the involvement may be different for a basic science researcher who works in a laboratory setting than for a social science researcher whose lab is the community where study participants live. The topics, materials, and tools of the social scientist, when used in the context of the participatory action paradigm, already expose that researcher to the values and attitudes of an intended audience, expected uses for the new knowledge, and the context for its uptake. One could argue that this would place the social scientist in an excellent position to engage in effective knowledge exchange with potential users of that knowledge.

However, the very nature of new knowledge in social science research adds a complexity to planning for and anticipating its uptake and use. The new knowledge often reveals the complexities or nuances in human perspectives and behaviours. After all, the nature of qualitative research is to uncover the multiple perspectives inherent in the human condition. Trying to turn this breadth and diversity of information to 'useable' knowledge or an evidence base for decision-making in patient care is a significant challenge. This is a critical challenge we must confront in the field of qualitative and participatory action research if we are to achieve effective knowledge exchange.

There are multiple areas of expertise required to be successful in this process of knowledge exchange. And clearly, there is a need for partnerships. Effective partnerships are needed with experts in social marketing, adult education, diffusion theory, and communications just to work through getting the message right and selecting the appropriate format for that message. One would need to have partnerships with representatives of the intended audience to understand the arena in which the knowledge was to be used and how it could be used within the scope of the role and responsibilities. Understanding if systems-change would be needed and how to orchestrate that change is best articulated by those who know the system. Lavis et al. (2003, p. 222) outline five key questions that applied research organizations could use as an organizing framework for knowledge transfer:

1 What should be transferred to decision-makers (the message)?
2 To whom should research knowledge be transferred (the target audience)?
3 By whom should the research knowledge be transferred (the messenger)?

4 How should research knowledge be transferred (the knowledge transfer processes and communication infrastructure)?
5 With what effect should research knowledge be transferred (evaluation)?

One could imagine that with various audiences, the details in the answers to these questions would vary: general public/service recipients (e.g., citizens, patients, and clients), service providers (e.g., clinicians), managerial decision-makers (i.e., managers in hospitals, community organizations, and private businesses), and policy decision-makers at the federal, provincial/regional, or municipal/local level (Power & Eisenberg, 1998). Within one study, there could be several messages for different audiences that each demand a different approach.

As an example, the OBCCRI work conducted with women living in low-income situations has a key message that 'having cancer costs.' But who needs to hear that message and act on it – Social workers in the field who help with applications for funding support? Chief executive officers of cancer centres who would be in a position to implement a new support program for low-resourced patients? Insurance company field officers or executives who determine approaches for reimbursement of claims? I suggest they all need to hear the message about patient needs and challenges, but that the approaches for informing each target audience and recommending specific action steps for them need to be tailored. What is perceived as meaningful by one audience may not be by another. What will catch and keep the attention of one will be different than another.

Another example concerns a message that comes from looking across all the OBCCRI studies – there is a need for more information and support for patients during and following treatment for cancer. Patients are not receiving the kind and amount of information and support that they feel they need. Survivors still face many challenges and have numerous questions. Who is the audience for that message? Does one go to advocacy groups and provide them with the stories and the data so that they can influence policy makers in various levels of government? Or should the information go to the directors of cancer centres or coordinators of supportive care in Ontario regional cancer groups, both of whom are charged with the responsibility of ensuring comprehensive cancer care is provided in their jurisdiction? Or does one take the information to peer and support groups in the community to provide evidence for them to use in their fundraising campaigns for money to enlarge their support programs for patients and families? Clearly, the message and intended use need to be linked to the relevant audience.

Without a doubt, it could be argued that all these directions make a great deal of sense to pursue. Very likely, all of them have merit. For any one project, there could be a variety of audiences who ought to hear about the results. Yet there are finite energy and resources for this work. From a researcher perspective, one has to choose where to place emphasis and energy. One has to determine how to make that decision. Each project team will likely have to debate this point in the context of their work and what is achievable.

Relationships

Everything I have read indicates to me that relationships are a key to successful knowledge transfer. It is through relationships that action happens. And the stronger those relationships are, the easier it will be to work through them. One could argue, then, that the starting point for effective knowledge exchange is within the strongest relationships – ones where there is mutual respect, trust, and common (shared) agendas. If they do not exist, these relationships will need to be built as a first step in sharing research results that will ultimately make a difference. This is perhaps one of the most significant lessons from the work within OBCCRI.

As a research community, OBCCRI built strong relationships with a range of people and organizations. In turn, these individuals and organizations have their own networks and links with other agencies. These links and networks – established at the outset of the OBCCRI work and honed through the ways in which we conducted our work – are the starting points, the pathways, for successful knowledge exchange. Through dialogue and discussion, we can ensure that the research in which we engage is about relevant, meaningful topics to women with breast cancer. By working together we can sort out the right message, for the right audience, and the form that message needs to take. Together we can work out the anticipated best use for new knowledge, how that knowledge can influence and facilitate change, the best routes to reach the intended audience, and potential obstacles or barriers to success. Researchers need to be a part of the knowledge exchange process, but they require effective partnerships to make knowledge exchange a successful reality.

Challenges Ahead for Qualitative and Participatory
Action Researchers

Before I draw this chapter to a close, I want to step back from my position within the OBCCRI and look through another lens. I served as provincial coordinator of Supportive Care for Cancer Care Ontario for ten years (1995–2005) and am currently Chair of the ReBalance Focus Action Group of the Canadian Strategy for Cancer Control. I am also currently serving as president of the International Society of Nurses in Cancer Care. These positions offer the opportunity to see the type of research conducted by OBCCRI within the context of a larger landscape. This 'big picture' lens allows me to say without reservation that this type of research is important to the future of cancer care as well as healthcare. Taken together, its focus, its populations, its communities, its approaches, its way of being in the world, place it in a niche where it has a vital contribution to make. In particular, the type of work conducted by OBCCRI is very important and necessary for improving the care of cancer patients and their family members. It is work that must be launched, inserted, and embedded within the cancer system in meaningful and relevant ways if we are to change the experiences that patients and families undergo.

In each of the roles I hold, I have had the opportunity to hear about, and see, firsthand, the impact of a cancer diagnosis and its treatment. It is not simply a physical impact. There are social, psychological, emotional, and spiritual consequences as well. It is a life event that brings irrevocable changes. Repeatedly, patients and survivors have told us that good (effective, supportive) communication with healthcare professionals and access to relevant information and support are critically important to their coping throughout the cancer experience. Yet, over and over again, observations have been made that there is variation from region to region, jurisdiction to jurisdiction, in the availability of and access to supportive care services. By definition, supportive care is the provision of the necessary services, as defined by those living with or affected by cancer, to meet their physical, informational, emotional, psychological, social, spiritual, and practical needs during the pre-diagnostic, diagnostic, treatment, and follow-up phases, encompassing issues of survivorship, palliative care, and bereavement (Fitch, 2000).

The knowledge uncovered through qualitative and participatory research can help us understand the experience from the person's perspective. It can help us comprehend the pathways to developing approaches and programs that are relevant and appropriate to patients and survivors and their families. The voices that emerge from this type of research can bring remarkable wisdom to the discussion about quality of life, quality of care, and improvements in care delivery.

The ReBalance Focus Action Group of the Canadian Strategy on Cancer Control was established to provide leadership directed towards changing the focus of cancer care so that patients' needs are better served. The establishment of this group signals that Canadian cancer control leaders have acknowledged the importance of cancer care being responsive to the full range of needs experienced by patients and survivors. They saw the desirability of changing the focus of the cancer care system from tumour-centred care to patient-centred care, and from being predominantly bio-medical in approach to being bio-psychosocial in approach. Other nations have also incorporated supportive and person-centred care as key components in their cancer control strategies (i.e., United Kingdom, New South Wales in Australia), and patient and survivor considerations are being incorporated into many of the other cancer control planning processes of other countries (International Conference on Cancer Control, 2005). These trends are very encouraging and hold hope for future change. However, they need to be informed by the full range of research evidence.

In moving our efforts forward to have the discoveries of qualitative and participatory action research embraced and utilized, we need to face the current realities in healthcare delivery and find ways to work effectively in light of these realities. We need to be ever cognizant of the trends and priorities that are influencing program budget planning or allocations. It is easy for the fiscally strapped system to be preoccupied with costly chemotherapeutic agents, lengthy waiting times for surgery, and limited access to radiation treatment, with little parallel consideration for patients' psychosocial distress, financial burden, or spiritual turmoil. Our challenge is to find the communication strategies that will garner attention to the evidence from our work and influence the processes of decision-making.

Additionally, beliefs about what constitutes science, research, measurement, and outcomes are still predominantly embedded in a paradigm of analytical positivism. The attitude towards embracing a wide range of evidence, and seeing that different types of evidence are needed for different purposes, is growing slowly. There is still a need for education about the use of specific evidence in appropriate and particular ways, and how different types of evidence may necessitate different designs and approaches to data collection. For example, if I want to know which chemotherapeutic agent is most appropriate, with the least toxicities, for a certain type and stage of cancer I need evidence from a large sample Randomized Clinical Trial. But if I want to gain a deep understanding of patient feelings and experiences, I need evidence from a data collection manoeuvre that involves human interaction, exchange, and in-depth dialogue. In both instances, however, I want rigour and excellence in the methods applied to generate the evidence. One might argue that lack of exposure to the naturalistic paradigm and lack of understanding about its philosophical basis could be key stumbling blocks for some cancer care providers and policy makers. Many have not had the opportunity to learn about the philosophical foundations and appropriate methods in qualitative work, or how the resulting knowledge can inform care delivery activities.

The past fifteen years have seen an encouraging growth in the Canadian community of psychosocial and behavioural researchers (including supportive care and palliative care), and the development of a credible body of research knowledge. There is a growing openness to multiple methods and methodologies, as well as appreciation for different types of evidence. Some of the key cancer research funding organizations (i.e., National Cancer Institute of Canada, Canadian Institutes of Health Research) are beginning to offer opportunities in topic areas such as palliative care, health services research, and knowledge transfer. The challenge for us is to take advantage of these opportunities and continue to grow the field.

Concluding Comments

In drawing this chapter and book to a close, I see two major considerations ahead for qualitative and participatory action researchers as we promote our research results to make a difference in patient care or policy. First, there is a challenge concerning the nature of the work and the fact that it may not be readily evident how it can be used. We need to be proactive in helping others understand how the work can be used. I can see that there are several questions we need to be asking about our results: What is the expectation for 'use' regarding a specific piece of qualitative work? When has it been used to its full extent or used enough? What do we want to achieve with a particular result? Is it to increase awareness? Is it to change a particular practice? Is it to stimulate a different approach in how patients are assessed or in the dialogue with patients? Does it mean we have a new intervention to offer? When is qualitative research ready for sharing? Should all of it be shared for the purpose of 'use' in the clinical world?

I am not convinced that all clinical practitioners or policy makers listening to narratives from patient experience research or presentations from rigorous qualitative research projects would know immediately how to 'use' the research findings in their practice. And who is best to identify the most beneficial use of the knowledge – the researcher or the potential user? I believe there needs to be more dialogue and discussion about this notion of 'use' of research results, such as ours, in the world of cancer care. As qualitative researchers, we face the reality that practitioners, decision-makers, and policy makers live in work environments where there are growing numbers of patients, increasing complexities in treatment procedures, and seemingly ever-decreasing resources. Sorting through research findings to determine how to make use of them within their clinical environment or community setting may not be their priority.

The other major challenge I see relates to the nature of the change needed if one really *listens* to the results from work such as OBCCRI has presented in this book. For me, the stories uncovered through the efforts of OBCCRI imply the need for significant systemic change in our cancer system. This change is not just a tweak here or there, a new program in one or two cancer settings, but a fundamental change in how we 'do cancer care.' This is a change that cannot be accomplished by one discipline or one jurisdiction. The change will need collaborative efforts and shared understanding about what is to be accomplished. Phrases such as 'patient-centred care,' 'person-centred care,' 'survivor driven programs,' and 'interventions tailored to the individual' are used to describe what is needed in our cancer care system. Understanding what these phrases truly mean and how to achieve them in a clinical setting is important. I believe that through rigorous qualitative and participatory action research we can begin to understand what these concepts mean and how to enact them in authentic ways. How do we tailor care for a black woman living with breast cancer, for a young woman confronting recurrent breast disease, or for a woman living in a low-resource situation? The results of the work presented in this book give us insight regarding what these phrases could mean and what might be required in order to make them real for some women. The methods give us models we could use in learning together with other communities – what do the phrases really mean for women living with ovarian cancer, men living with prostate cancer, or those struggling with lung cancer?

From my perspective, there is much yet to do. The work has really just begun. And although the road may be difficult, filled with challenges and complexities, I believe the journey will be worth making.

REFERENCES

Best, A. (2006). *Integrating knowledge strategies: New models for more effective action*. Paper presentation at the OBCCRI Workshop on Knowledge Exchange, Toronto, February.

Blasi, Z.D., Harkness, E., Ernst, E., Georgiou, A., & Kleijnen, J. (2001). Influence of context effects on health outcomes: A systematic review. *Lancet, 357*, 757–62.

Canadian Institutes of Health. (2002). Knowledge translation fact sheet. Available from www.cihr-irsc.gc.ca/e/26574.html

Canadian Strategy for Cancer Control. Rebalance Focus Action Group priorities. (2004). Available from www.cancercontrol.org/cscc/priorities_rfpage.html

Estabrooks, C.A. (1999). The conceptual structure of research utilization. *Research in Nursing & Health, 22*(3), 203–16.

Eveland, J.D. (1986). Diffusion, technology transfer and implementation. *Knowledge, 8*, 303–22.

Fitch, M. (2000). Supportive care for cancer patients. *Hospital Quarterly, 3*(4), 39–6.

Gabbey, J., & le May, A. (2004). Evidence based guidelines or collectively constructed 'mindlines'? Ethnographic study of knowledge management in primary care. *British Medical Journal, 329*, 1013–17.

Graham, I.D., & Logan, J. (2004). Translating research – innovations in knowledge transfer and continuity of care. *Canadian Journal of Nursing Research, 36*(2), 89–103.

Greenhalgh, T., Robert, G., MacFarlane, F., Bate, P., & Kyriakidou, O. (2004). Diffusion of innovations in service organizations: Systematic review and recommendations. *Milbank Quarterly, 82*, 581–629.

Grol, R. (1997). Beliefs and evidence in changing clinical practice. *British Medical Journal, 315*, 418–21.

Grol, R., & Grimshaw, J. (2003). From best evidence to best practice: Effective implementation of change in patients' care. *Lancet, 362*, 1225–30.

Grunfeld, E., Zitzelsberger, L., Hayter, C., Berman, N., Cameron, R., Evans,

W.K., & Stern, H. (2004) The role of knowledge translation for cancer control in Canada. *Chronic Diseases in Canada, 25*(2), 1–6.

International Congress on Cancer Control. (2005). Proceedings available at http://www.cancercontrol.org/cscc/archive_2005.html

Landry, R., Amara, N., & Lamari, M. (2002). Climbing the ladder of research utilization: Evidence from social research. *Science Communication, 22,* 396–422.

Larsen, J.K. (1980). Knowledge utilization: What is it? *Knowledge: Creation, Diffusion, Utilization, 1,* 421–43.

Lavis, J.N., Robertson, D., Woodside, J., McLeod, C., Abelson, J., & The Knowledge Transfer Study Group. (2003). How can research organizations more effectively transfer research knowledge to decision-makers? *The Milbank Quarterly, 81*(2) 221–48.

Logan, J., & Graham, I.D. (1998). Toward a comprehensive interdisciplinary model of health care research use. *Science Communication, 20,* 227–46.

Lomas, J. (1993). Diffusion, dissemination, and implementation: Who should do what? *Annals of New York Academy of Science, 703,* 226–35.

Lomas, J. (2000). Connecting research and policy. Available from http://www.isuma.net/v01n01/index_e.shtml

McCall, D.S., Rootman, I., & Bayley, D. (2005). International School Health Network: An informal network for advocacy and knowledge exchange. *Promotional Health, 12*(3), 173–7.

Montague, T. (2006). Patient-provider partnerships in health care: Enhancing knowledge translation and improving outcomes. *Healthcare Papers, 7*(2), 56–61.

National Center for the Dissemination of Disability Research. (1996). A review of the literature on dissemination and knowledge utilization. NCDDR. www.ncddr.org/du/products/review/index.html

Oxman, A.D. (1995) No magic bullets: A systematic review of 102 trials of interventions to improve professional practice. *Canadian Medical Association Journal, 153,* 1423–31.

Power, E.J., & Eisenberg, J.M. (1998). Are we ready to use cost-effectiveness analysis in health care decision making? A health services research challenge for clinicians, patients, health care systems, and public policy. *Medical Care, 36*(5 Suppl.), MS10–147.

Rogers, E.M. (2002). The nature of technology transfer. *Science Communication, 23,* 323–41.

Rogers, E.M. (2003). *Diffusion of innovations* (5th ed.). New York: Free Press.

University of Toronto. (2001). As adapted from the CIHR definition. Definition available at http://www.ktp.utoronto.ca/whatisktp/definition/

Recommended Sources For Further Reading

Qualitative Research: General

Alvesson, M., & Skoldberg, K. (2000). *Reflexive methodology: New vistas for qualitative research.* London: Sage.

Bazeley, P. (2007). *Qualitative data analysis with NVivo.* London: Sage.

Berg, B. (2007). *Qualitative research methods for the social sciences* (6th ed.). Boston: Pearson Allyn Bacon.

Creswell, J. (2003). *Research design: Qualitative, quantitative, and mixed method approaches* (2nd ed.). Thousand Oaks, CA: Sage.

Krueger, R., & Casey, M. (2000). *Focus groups: A practical guide for applied research* (3rd ed.). Newbury Park, CA: Sage.

Lincoln, Y., & Guba, E. (1985). *Naturalistic inquiry.* Beverly Hills, CA: Sage.

Mason, J. (1996). *Qualitative researching.* Thousand Oaks, CA: Sage.

Morse, J., & Richards, L. (2002). *Read me first for a user's guide to qualitative methods.* Thousand Oaks, CA: Sage.

Morse, J., Swanson, J., & Kuzel, A. (Eds.). (2001). *The nature of qualitative evidence.* Thousand Oaks, CA: Sage.

Nagy Hesse-Biber, S., & Leavy, P. (Eds.). (2003). *Approaches to qualitative research: A reader on theory and practice.* Oxford: Oxford University Press.

Rubin, H., & Rubin, I. (1995). *Qualitative interviewing: The art of hearing data.* Thousand Oaks, CA: Sage.

Community-Based Participatory Action Research (CBPAR)

Kirby, S., Greaves, L., & Reid, C. (2006). *Experience, research, social change: Methods beyond the mainstream.* Toronto: Broadview Press.

Maguire, P. (1987). *Doing participatory research: A feminist approach.* Amherst, MA: Center for International Education.

Moosa-Mitha, M. (2005). Situating anti-oppressive theories within critical and difference-centred perspectives. In I. Brown & S. Strega (Eds.), *Research as resistance: Critical, indigenous, and anti-oppressive approaches* (pp. 237–54). Toronto: Canadian Scholars' Press.

Reitsma-Street, M., & Brown, L. (2004). Community action research. In W. Carroll (Ed.), *Critical strategies for social research* (pp. 303–19). Toronto: Canadian Scholars' Press.

Ristock, J., & Pennell, J. (1996). *Community research as empowerment: Feminist links, postmodern interruptions.* Toronto: Oxford University Press.

St. Denis, V. (2004). Community-based participatory research: Aspects of the concept relevant for practice. In W. Carroll (Ed.), *Critical strategies for social research* (pp. 292–302). Toronto: Canadian Scholars' Press.

Whitmore, E. (2002). They listened to what we had to say: Emancipatory evaluation. In I. Shaw & N. Gould (Eds.), *Qualitative inquiry* (pp. 79–91). Thousand Oaks, CA: Wadsworth.

Community Organizing/Community Development

Minkler, M. (Ed.). (2005). *Community organizing and community building for health* (2nd ed.). New Jersey: Rutgers University Press.

Critical Analysis

Allen, D., & Cloyes, K. (2005). The language of 'experience' in nursing research. *Nursing Inquiry, 12*(2), 98–105.

Foucault, M. (1980). *Power/knowledge: Selected interviews and other writings, 1972–1977.* C. Gordon (Ed. and Trans.). New York: Pantheon Books.

Foucault, M. (1982). The subject and power. *Critical Inquiry, 8*: 777–95.

Feminist Research Methods

Lather, P. (1988). Feminist perspectives on empowering research methodologies. *Women's Studies International Forum, 11*(6), 569–81.

Nagy Hesse-Biber, S. (Ed.). (2007). *Handbook of feminist research theory and praxis.* Thousand Oaks, CA: Sage.

Reinharz, S. (1992). *Feminist methods in social research.* New York: Oxford University Press.

Ribbens, J., & Edwards, R. (Eds.). (1998). *Feminist dilemmas in qualitative research: Public knowledge and private lives.* London: Sage (reprinted in 2000 and 2006).

Ethnography

Madison, S. (2005). *Critical ethnography: Method, ethics, and performance.* Thousand Oaks, CA: Sage.

Discourse Analysis

Chouliaraki, L., & Fairclough, N. (2004). The critical analysis of discourse. In W. Carroll (Ed.), *Critical strategies for social research* (pp. 262–75). Toronto: Canadian Scholars' Press.

Parker, I. (2004). Discovering discourses, tackling texts. In W. Carroll (Ed.), *Critical strategies for social research.* Toronto: Canadian Scholars' Press.

Phillips, L., & Jørgensen, W. (2002). *Discourse analysis as theory and method.* London: Sage.

Narrative Analysis

Chambon, A. (1994). The dialogical analysis of case materials. In E. Sherman & W. Reid (Eds.), *Qualitative research in social work* (pp. 205–15). New York: Columbia University Press.

Lieblich, A., Tuval-Mashiach, R., & Zilber, T. (1998). *Narrative research: Reading, analysis, and interpretation.* Thousand Oaks, CA: Sage.

Grounded Theory

Charmaz, K. (2003). Grounded theory. In S. Nagy Hesse-Biber & P. Leavy (Eds.), *Approaches to qualitative research: A reader on theory and practice* (pp. 496–521). Oxford: Oxford University Press.

Mauthner, N., & Doucet, A. (1998). Reflections on a Voice-centred relational method: Analysing maternal and domestic voices. In J. Ribbens & R. Edwards (Eds.), *Feminist dilemmas in qualitative research* (pp. 9–36). Thousand Oaks, CA: Sage.

Representation

Alldred, P. (1998). Ethnography and discourse analysis: Dilemmas in representing the voices of children. In J. Ribbens & R. Edwards (Eds.), *Feminist dilemmas in qualitative research: Public knowledge and private lives* (pp. 147–70). Thousand Oaks, CA: Sage.

Borland, K. (2003). 'That's not what I said': Interpretive conflict in oral narrative research. In S. Nagy Hesse-Biber & P. Leavy (Eds.), *Approaches to qualitative research: A reader on theory and practice*. Oxford: Oxford University Press.

Fine, M., Weis, L., Weseen, S., & Wong, L. (2003). For whom? Qualitative research, representations and social responsibilities. In N. Denzin & Y. Lincoln (Eds.), *The landscape of qualitative research: Theories and issues* (2nd ed.) (pp. 167–207). Thousand Oaks, CA: Sage.

Garman, N., & Piantanida, M. (Eds.). (2006). *The authority to imagine: The struggle toward representation in dissertation writing*. New York: P. Lang.

Social Justice

Fassin, D. (2001). Culturalism as ideology. In C.M. Obermeyer (Ed.), *Cultural perspectives on reproductive health* (pp. 300–17). Oxford: Oxford University Press.

Freire, P. (1973). *Pedagogy of the oppressed*. New York: Seabury Press.

Goldberg, D. (1993). *Racist culture, philosophy and the politics of meaning*. Oxford: Blackwell.

Gunaratnam, Y. (2003). *Researching 'race' and ethnicity: Methods, knowledge and power*. London: Sage.

Kumashiro, K. (2004). *Against common sense: Teaching and learning toward social justice*. New York: Routledge Falmer.

Lewis, G. (2000). *Race, gender, social welfare: Encounters in a postcolonial society*. Cambridge: Polity Press.

Malat, J. (2006). Expanding research on the racial disparity in medical treatment with ideas from sociology. *Health: An Interdisciplinary Journal for the Social Study of Health, Illness and Medicine, 10*(3), 303–21.

Knowledge Transfer

Baines, D. (2007). The case for catalytic validity: building health and safety through knowledge transfer. *Policy and Practice in Health and Safety, 5*(1), 75–89.

CIHR Institute of Population and Public Health; Canadian Population Health Initative. (2006). *Moving population and public health knowledge into action: A casebook of knowledge translation stories*.

Estabrooks, C., Thompson, D., Lovely, J., & Hofmeyer, A. (2006). A guide to knowledge translation theory. *Journal of Continuing Education in the Health Professions, 26*(1), 25–36.

Graham, I.D., Logan, J., Harrison, M.B., Straus, S.E., Tetroe, J., Caswell, W., et al. (2006). Lost in knowledge translation: Time for a map? *Journal of Continuing Education in the Health Professions, 26*(1), 13–24.

Grimshaw, J., Shirran, L., Thomas, R., et al. (2001). Changing provider behavior: An overview of systematic reviews of interventions. *Medical Care, 39*(8, Suppl. 2), II2–II45.

Quantitative Research

Babbie, E. (2007). *The practice of social research* (11th ed.). Belmont, CA: Wadsworth.

Neuman, L. (2006). *Social research methods: Qualitative and quantitative approaches* (6th ed.). Boston: Allyn & Bacon.

Glossary of Terms

Community-based participatory action research (CBPAR) is a collaborative process that involves members of relevant communities at every stage of the research. It engages community members in defining and understanding problems, as well as devising strategies to address these problems through research. CBPAR researchers attempt to ensure that participants' perspectives guide the formation and the analysis of research. This occurs by soliciting feedback from participants and incorporating their responses in analyses and reports. Community members are invested in the dissemination and use of research findings and ultimately in the improvement of health and quality of life. There is a growing recognition of the effectiveness of this type of research within health services, particularly for disadvantaged or underrepresented groups.

Dissemination is the process of making research widely available to others wherever possible in appropriate formats. Dissemination activities range from giving local presentations, workshops, seminars, and displays to publishing research results in academic journals and community newsletters.

Knowledge translation (KT) refers to the entire process encompassing knowledge creation, dissemination, interpretation, and the facilitation of research impact and uptake. These activities include the myriad relationships formed among researchers, community members, and decision-makers and between those who create knowledge and those who apply knowledge. At OBCCRI, we have adopted the Canadian Institutes of Health Research (CIHR) definition of knowledge translation.

LGBTT. An acronym for: lesbian, gay, bi-sexual, transsexual, and transgender communities.

Marginalized groups are those that are socially excluded based on systems such as racism, economic discrimination, sexism, and homophobia. People can be marginalized through financial disadvantage, mental or physical disability, culture, gender, religion, age, or race. Hence, access to healthcare is an issue affecting vulnerable groups whose needs are often sensitive and specific. Research with marginalized groups is concerned with understanding barriers to equal access, and with bringing the needs of underrepresented people to the awareness of healthcare providers, policy makers, and the general public.

Mixed methods research involves both qualitative (e.g., interviews) and quantitative (e.g., questionnaires) approaches. 'Mixing' might be within a single study or among several studies in a program of inquiry. This type of research has the potential to expand our understanding of a phenomenon; for example, interviews with individual women may provide insight about the reasons for statistically low attendance in a particular support service. Mixed methods approaches are becoming more common in various social and behavioural science disciplines, including education and health.

Psychosocial oncology is concerned with helping patients and families maintain emotional well-being and cope with the stresses associated with a cancer diagnosis and treatment. It encompasses issues aside from the medical treatment of cancer, such as psychological distress and social barriers to care.

Psychosocial research in oncology examines the emotional, psychological, and social impact that cancer has on patients and their families and carers. Some questions with which psychosocial research is generally concerned include: How do people react to a cancer diagnosis? How does cancer affect a person's daily life? Why do some patients decide not to finish their treatment? How do families react to a relative's cancer diagnosis? What are the barriers to care for some individuals or groups in society? Psychosocial research examines the role of support services, asking, for example: Do cancer patients live longer or is their quality of life better if they receive support during their disease? It also attempts to recommend new and better modes of doctor-patient communication and service delivery.

Qualitative research is concerned with understanding the nature of phenomena by paying close attention to individuals, groups, and their experiences. Quantitative research, on the other hand, seeks measurements of phenomena, for instance, 'What percentage of people do one thing or another?' Qualitative research can be useful for answering questions about 'why' a particular event, phenomenon, or issue exists. Qualitative research attempts to place events and phenomena in context, considering the complexity of social life. Qualitative methods include in-depth interviews, focus groups, observation of groups or events, and textual analysis. As a result, qualitative research produces large amounts of data in the form of transcripts and observational field-notes, and involves time-consuming and intensive preparation and analysis. Qualitative research is particularly suited to understanding the psychosocial issues of cancer patients and helping develop potential solutions in order to improve practice.

Quality of life. As cancer treatments are improving, more and more patients are recovering from this disease or living longer. Quality of life refers to how a patient's physical and psychological state affects his or her overall well-being and enjoyment of everyday life.

Supportive care is the care given to improve the coping ability and quality of life of those diagnosed with cancer by addressing the psychological, social, economic, and spiritual problems related to cancer or its treatment.

Contributors

Stephanie Austin is currently working as senior policy analyst at the Bureau of Women's Health and Gender Analysis at Health Canada. Stephanie holds a PhD in psychology and completed a Social Sciences and Humanities Research Council Post-doctoral Research Fellowship with the Ontario Breast Cancer Community Research Initiative in 2004 conducting studies on the psychosocial dimensions of marginalized women's experiences of breast cancer. Stephanie has maintained her connections to community-based action research since she co-founded POWER Camp, recently renamed Girls Action Foundation, an innovative program addressing equity and health issues for and with adolescent girls (see www.girlsaction.ca for details). She is an action-oriented and strategic thinker whose greatest strength lies in building effective collaborative networks. She intends to have a vibrant career where she can use her leadership skills to help design and implement innovative policy and research to enhance social inclusion, social cohesion, and equity in health in Canada.

Emerance Baker is an urban mixed-blood Mohawk/Cayuga-Hungarian. She currently serves as the University of Waterloo's Aboriginal Services Coordinator. Emerance's social sciences field of study in her undergraduate and graduate degrees specialized in women's health, the sociology of cancer prevention, research ethics and methodology, and Indigenous knowledge sharing. Emerance continued her work in the field of women's health with the Cancer Survivors and Healing Arts Pilot Project in Newfoundland, with the CIHR Aboriginal Women's Cancer Care Project out of Wilfrid Laurier University, and with Cancer Care Ontario's Community Capacity Building Projects. Emerance would like to thank 'the women and families who trusted me to share their stories more widely in the hopes of building understanding and compassion.' Emerance has four wonderful children and a husband who shares her commitment and passion for this community.

Lisa Barnoff is an associate professor in the School of Social Work at Ryerson University. Her research and writing explores the implementation of anti-oppression practices in social service agencies and on processes of anti-oppression organizational change. Lisa was also involved in the Lesbians and Breast Cancer Project, which explored lesbians' experiences with cancer and cancer care. Lisa's teaching areas include social work theory and practice, violence against women, family violence, sexual diversity, and anti-oppressive social work.

Falia Damianakis was with the Ontario Breast Cancer Community Research Initiative as a community advisory member from 2001 until 2006. As a psychotherapist, educator-trainer, and health advocate, Falia has supported individuals and families facing life-threatening illness, loss, and grief since 1995. She has developed and implemented peer support programming for newly diagnosed women and breast cancer survivors at Willow, facilitated groups for people with cancer and their caregivers, and designed and led workshops to train facilitators, counsellors and volunteers. Falia's past diagnoses with cancer inform her understanding of the issues and concerns shared by those living with cancer. Drawing on her background as an artist and her experience in project development, she coordinated the production of a play about breast cancer, early detection, and the experiences of immigrant women with the healthcare system. Falia is interested in the use of creative forms of expression to raise awareness and engage in dialogue to effect personal and social change.

Margaret I. Fitch was a co-founder and director of OBCCRI from 2001 to 2007. She has research interests in patient and survivor experiences with cancer and coping with the many challenges this illness brings into individuals' lives. She has been highly involved at both national and international levels in cancer control planning initiatives. Dr. Fitch is currently the head of Oncology Nursing and Supportive Care at the Odette Cancer Centre and an associate professor at the Faculty of Nursing, University of Toronto.

Judy Gould is a research scientist and was the initiative director of the Ontario Breast Cancer Community Research Initiative (OBCCRI). She is also an assistant professor in the Department of Public Health Sciences at the University of Toronto. Her graduate training focused on Community and Social Psychology. Her work with the OBCCRI was focused on understanding the issues/needs of lower-income and young women who have experienced breast cancer. Additionally, in partnership with Dr. Sue Wilson from Ryerson University and Pamela Grassau from the OBCCRI, she implemented a qualitative and longitudinal exploration of how women understand spirituality in the context of having a breast cancer diagnosis.

Pamela Grassau is a PhD candidate in the Faculty of Social Work at the University of Toronto, and a sessional instructor in the School of Social Work at Carleton University. Pam was a research associate with the OBCCRI from 2001 to 2006. Pam's doctoral work focuses on relational narratives of breast cancer, specifically those between mothers and their adolescent daughters. Using qualitative and arts-based methods in this site, she engages openly and explicitly about 'difference' across experiences, identities, roles, and contexts. Other areas of interest are: community-based participatory research and social action, the application of intersectionality and anti-oppressive theory in health, and teaching and engaging with a range of research methods (from arts-based modalities, to working with qualitative software, to mixed-method designs). Pam strives to reflect and apply anti-oppressive practice frameworks in her social work practice, research, and teaching.

Ross Gray was a co-founder of OBCCRI and was co-director from 2001 to 2005. He is an associate professor in the Faculty of Medicine at the University of Toronto and is a psychologist in private practice. Known as an innovator in the representation of qualitative social science research, he initiated and performed in the research-based dramas *Handle with Care? Women Living with Metastatic Breast Cancer* and *No Big Deal?* about the issues facing men with prostate cancer and their partners. He is the author of more than one hundred academic papers, three books, and numerous articles for lay audiences.

Kara Griffin obtained her undergraduate degree in psychology from the University of Prince Edward Island and a master's degree in community psychology from Wilfrld Laurier University. She was research coordinator for the Ontario Breast Cancer Survivor Dragon Boat Study from 2002 to 2004. She is an experienced researcher in qualitative and community-based participatory research. Kara is currently a researcher in public health policy at the University of Toronto.

Sue Keller-Olaman trained as a social scientist in New Zealand (PhD level; psychology and preventive and social medicine). She currently works for the City of Hamilton, reviewing services and program areas across Public Health Services. Sue also holds an adjunct position at McMaster University (Health, Aging and Society) and undertakes consulting work. She completed post-doctoral research at McMaster University (Institute of Environment and Health). Sue has worked for both the Ontario Breast Cancer Community Research Initiative (OBCCRI) and the Ontario Breast Cancer Information Exchange Partnership (OBCIEP, now OBCEP). Sue's research interests include determinants of health, program evaluation and review, peer support, and environment-health relationships.

Patti McGillicuddy completed her undergraduate degrees in social work and in religious studies at McMaster University and a master's degree in social work at the University of Toronto majoring in community development and social planning. Patti is currently the interprofessional education leader and an education/research associate for Allied Health at the University Health Network in Toronto. Previously, Patti was the professional leader for social work at Sunnybrook HSC and at Women's College Hospital in Toronto, Ontario. She has an appointment at the University of Toronto, Social Work, and has developed and taught courses at Ryerson University in the Internationally Trained Social Workers Bridging Program. Within the past thirty-four years she has worked as a manager, clinician, program planner, policy developer, educator, and researcher in the areas of trauma, personal violence, mental health, cancer care, and women's health.

Terry Mitchell is an associate professor in the Department of Psychology at Wilfrid Laurier University and is the director of the Centre for Community Research, Learning, and Action. She received her PhD in community psychology from the University of Toronto and has dedicated her scholarly activities to developing and sharing skills in qualitative methods and community-based participatory research. Dr. Mitchell has been working with Aboriginal communities for over fifteen years. Her work investigates inequities in health and health services with attention to historical and political injustices that have resulted in intergenerational trauma. She is committed to advancing post-colonial critiques with attention to advocacy for individual and community healing.

Jennifer J. Nelson is the co-founder of Cardinal Consultants, which provides social science research services to a variety of professional and government agencies, including healthcare, law, and education. She is also affiliated with the University of Toronto as assistant professor in the Department of Public Health Sciences, where she is principal investigator on a SSHRC grant examining professional helping encounters across social inequalities. She completed her PhD at OISE/UT in sociology and equity studies in education in 2001. She is the author of *Razing Africville: A Geography of Racism* (University of Toronto Press, 2008).

Fran Odette is the program manager of the Women with Disabilities and Deaf Women's Program at Education Wife Assault. Fran's work in the violence against women movement has had a particular focus on issues impacting women with disabilities and deaf women. As an educator/trainer, 'access to services and inclusion to the/our community' are essential messages Fran hopes to leave with service providers and agencies in their own efforts to make the linkages needed to ensure greater access to services for all women. In 2004, Fran co-authored, with Cory Silverberg and Dr. Miriam Kaufman, *The Ultimate Guide to Sex and Disability – For All of Us Who Live with Disabilities, Chronic Pain and Illness* (Cleis Press).

Chris Sinding is an associate professor at McMaster University jointly appointed to the Department of Health, Aging and Society and the School of Social Work. Her research and teaching focus on health and social justice (or, more accurately/more often, illness and social injustice). Her current research is with and about people with cancer, their families, and supporters. She works in interpretive and critical traditions, foregrounding the meanings research participants assign to their experiences and interactions and examining their accounts with reference to health systems and broad patterns of domination and exclusion. She is interested in innovative – particularly arts-informed – knowledge exchange (both doing it, and taking it as an object of study).

Ann Wray Hampson (MEd, Counselling) is a counsellor with experience in private practice and group leadership. She has been associated with Wellspring, a support centre for patients, families, and health professionals, as a program developer, leader, and committee member. She has also participated in research projects related to issues of dealing with illness, loss, and change.

Index

Index 289